Praise for *Ethics for Psychothe*

T0260729

"Anderson and Handelsman have written a truly unique ethics book; one that will be of value to every new as well as seasoned psychotherapist in professions from social work to psychiatry. They write about professional ethics as a process of acculturation that requires the reader to consider themselves, their motivations, and their feelings about the ethical requirements of the professions. In order to facilitate the process of self-awareness, they provide a series of activities like journaling to help the professional continue to expand their awareness as they encounter topics like confidentiality or multiple relationships. Whether or not instructor chooses this book as a primary text, it should be a supplement to every course that is taught."

Karen Strohm Kitchener, Professor Emeritus, University of Denver

"This book is unique in my experience in that it encourages readers to reflect on their own ethical predispositions as they think about psychotherapy ethics. The book also helps students understand differences between being an ethical person and an ethical psychotherapist – a distinction that is difficult for most students, and many professionals, to appreciate. The authors' emphasis on helping readers know themselves as well as the professional ethical guidelines is an important advance over other ethics texts. The discussion of 'positive ethics' is also unique and helpful for professionals."

William E. Sobesky, Clinical Associate Professor of Psychiatry and Pediatrics, University of Colorado Health Sciences Center

"This excellent book for students or any professionals in psychotherapy and counseling is part of a welcome trend in ethics education that challenges students to strive for their highest ethical ideals. Anderson and Handelsman do far more than repeat rules and facts; they use the ethical acculturation model to encourage students to reflect on their professional identity and values. The book contains useful learning aides and exercises such as the ethics autobiography, the ethics journal, realistic vignettes, appendices, and useful charts. Anderson and Handelsman succeed in presenting their well considered perspectives on psychotherapy in a clear and personal style of writing. I highly recommend this book!"

Samuel Knapp, Director of Professional Affairs, Pennsylvania Psychological Association

"This book is interesting and engaging. A variety of scenarios and exercises make the process come alive for the reader and encourage self-assessment and self-reflection. As an instructor I think the text would generate many meaningful class discussions. It is easy-to-read and easy to follow."

Robin Lewis, Old Dominion University

"I really like this book....it approaches ethics in a manner that is hopeful, positive, but no-nonsense and thorough. I think it is one of the best integration of concepts around ethics and ethical decision-making processes that I have seen, and one of the most easily applied to a variety of levels of training. I also like the application of an acculturation model as a way to understand our initiation into the part of our profession that has to do with ethics, ethical decision-making, and ethical behavior."

Susan L. Prieto-Welch, Counseling Center Director, University of Notre Dame

To KK – mentor, colleague, and friend.

And JC – thank you! You are so good to me.

Sharon

To my mother, Eleanore Welsh. To my wife, Margie Krest.

And to all my teachers, including all my students.

Mitch

Ethics for Psychotherapists and Counselors

A Proactive Approach

Sharon K. Anderson
Colorado State University

Mitchell M. Handelsman
University of Colorado Denver

WILEY-BLACKWELL

A John Wiley & Sons, Ltd., Publication

This edition first published 2010
© 2010 Sharon K. Anderson and Mitchell M. Handelsman

Blackwell Publishing was acquired by John Wiley & Sons in February 2007. Blackwell's publishing program has been merged with Wiley's global Scientific, Technical, and Medical business to form Wiley-Blackwell.

Registered Office
John Wiley & Sons Ltd, The Atrium, Southern Gate, Chichester, West Sussex, PO19 8SQ, United Kingdom

Editorial Offices
350 Main Street, Malden, MA 02148-5020, USA
9600 Garsington Road, Oxford, OX4 2DQ, UK
The Atrium, Southern Gate, Chichester, West Sussex, PO19 8SQ, UK

For details of our global editorial offices, for customer services, and for information about how to apply for permission to reuse the copyright material in this book please see our website at www.wiley.com/wiley-blackwell.

The right of Sharon K. Anderson and Mitchell M. Handelsman to be identified as the authors of this work has been asserted in accordance with the Copyright, Designs and Patents Act 1988.

Library of Congress Cataloging-in-Publication Data

Anderson, Sharon K.
  Ethics for psychotherapists and counselors : a proactive approach/Sharon K. Anderson, Mitchell M. Handelsman.
    p. ; cm.
  Includes bibliographical references and index.
  ISBN 978-1-4051-7767-2 (hardcover: alk. paper) – ISBN 978-1-4051-7766-5 (pbk. : alk. paper) 1. Psychotherapists–Professional ethics. 2. Counselors–Professional ethics. I. Handelsman, Mitchell M. II. Title.
  [DNLM: 1. Psychotherapy–ethics. 2. Counseling–ethics. WM 420 A549e 2010]
  RC455.2.E8A53 2010
  616.89'14–dc22
                                                          2009009595

A catalogue record for this book is available from the British Library.

Set in Palatino 10/13 pt by SPi Publisher Services, Pondicherry, India

1   2010

Contents

About the Authors

Sharon K. Anderson received her Ph.D. in counselling psychology from the University of Denver. She has taught in masters level counselling program at Colorado State University since 1994. As a professor, she teaches the professional ethics and legal issues course and supervises practicum and internship experiences for master level counsellors. For several years, Sharon delivered state approved jurisprudence workshops to psychotherapists from many disciplines seeking state licensure. She herself is a licensed psychologist. During her time as faculty, Sharon has published 2 books, 10 book chapters, and 17 articles.

Mitchell M. Handelsman received his Ph.D. in clinical psychology from the University of Kansas. He has taught psychology at the University of Colorado Denver since 1982. He was an APA Congressional Science Fellow during 1989–1990, and in 2003–2004 he was president of the Rocky Mountain Psychological Association. He is a licensed psychologist and a Fellow of the American Psychological Association. In addition, he has won the CASE (Council for the Advancement and Support of Education) Colorado Professor of the Year Award and APA's Division 2 Teaching Award. He has served on numerous professional ethics committees, and has chaired the Colorado Psychological Association Ethics Committee.

Preface

Becoming an ethical psychotherapist or counselor is more than memorization of rules – it is a journey. We wrote this book to help students and practitioners navigate this journey toward a professional identity in a way that integrates their personal ethics and values with the professional ethics and traditions of psychotherapy and counseling.

Our book presents a variety of discussions, case scenarios, thought exercises, and writing assignments to (a) introduce readers to all the major ethical issues in psychotherapy, including boundaries, confidentiality, informed consent, supervision, and terminating therapy; (b) help readers explore their own moral and ethical backgrounds, personal values, ethical thinking, cultural awareness, and professional goals; and (c) take a proactive and preventive approach to applying ethics to every facet of their professional behavior.

The book can be used as a primary or ancillary text for ethics courses in all the mental health fields. It can also be used as a supplemental text for courses in professional issues, psychotherapy methods, counseling theories and techniques, and survey courses in clinical and counseling psychology, social work, counseling, and marital and family therapy.

Because this book focuses on the basic aspects of professional identity and ethical reasoning skills, it will be useful to readers over time as they readjust their professional identities in reaction to inevitable changes in life situations, professional positions, laws/regulations, and ethics codes.

After years of discussion – between ourselves and with colleagues and students – about what it means to be ethically excellent, not just aware of how to stay out of ethical trouble, we decided to write a book that takes a unique approach. Students will find the book engaging, positive in its approach, and respectful of their backgrounds. We invite them to become active explorers, not passive recipients of disembodied rules and laws.

We also wrote this book to help us teach our own courses, and for our fellow instructors who may be new to teaching ethical issues as an entire course or part of a course. Instructors will find that they can organize class discussions and assignments around the exercises and vignettes from the chapters, or they can use the book to supplement their own methods and materials.

We wish to thank many people who have been involved in the long journey we've taken since our initial conversations about an ethics book. Our agent, Neil Salkind of Studio B, was instrumental in helping us conceive of this book in its present form and in encouraging us to undertake the project. Our editor, Christine Cardone, has been consistently supportive and instructive – providing just the right amount of guidance to bring this project to fruition. Thanks to Sam Knapp and Michael Gottlieb for their essential work on the ethical acculturation model, and to Allison Bashe for her work on the ethics autobiography. We thank those who provided such careful reviews of this text: R. Rocco Cottone, Robin Lewis, Susan Prieto-Welch, William Sobesky, and Rita Sommers-Flanagan. The following people have provided valuable assistance and feedback to us regarding previous iterations of the book: Tamar Ares, Bill Briggs, Pam Daniel, Pam Fritzler, Sharon Hamm, Susan Heitler, Mark Kirchhofer, Teresa Kostenbauer, Margie Krest, Amos Martinez, Natalie Meinerz, Amber Reed, and Deb Wescott.

Any imperfections that remain in the book, of course, are our responsibility alone.

Introduction

Imagine, if you would, sitting at a first-row table at a psychotherapist comedy club. You'd probably hear something like this from one of the bright young performers:

"What's the deal with becoming a psychotherapist? I mean, really! I figured the ethical issues – the issues of right and wrong – would be easy. Don't date your clients, keep their interests at the top of the list, be helpful, have nice furniture. But noooo!! Learning to be an ethical psychotherapist feels like going through the security lines at the airport! You can't do this, you can't do that, you can't bring that with you, and you can only bring so much of this. And then … there's this thing about how people start to treat you. I thought I would have years to learn all this stuff about being ethical. But, *nooo*! I mean I just started graduate school and right away friends and family members start treating me differently – like I'm Sigmund Freud or Dr Phil. I mean they want me to solve their problems. The first day of graduate school, right? I haven't even paid tuition or read the syllabus and when I get home my sister-in-law is there in my apartment asking how she should raise her kid! I go out to get some air and think about all her questions and my friend who lives on the floor below me asks me what I've been up to. I tell him that I've started graduate school to become a therapist and he tells me about his crazy sister – and asks if I have any time to "fix" her! My aunt calls up and says, 'Listen, call your cousin Marty and tell him he needs to see a shrink. He'll listen to you now.' I don't know how to respond to any of these pleas!"

Some audience members, mostly trainees, might not get the humor – or the reality behind the humor – in these stories because they don't see the ethical problems inherent in them. Why doesn't our young performer just see his friend's sister for treatment? Other members of the audience, mostly beginning therapists, might giggle and sigh at the same time because they understand the ethical dimensions and the situations are all too familiar. They recognize that psychotherapists face ethical decisions every day. How are new professionals to know the right things to do and to discern right and wrong professional behavior? Older, more experienced therapists among the audience members might shake their heads because they know that ethical situations, dilemmas, and decisions do not go away and often become more complex over the course of their careers. Of course, our young comedian can't tell the best stories – about clients – because of confidentiality.

Our book will have little impact on the fantasy psychotherapy-comedy club business, but it will help you in your journey toward becoming an ethical professional. We have written this book for all students of psychotherapy and counseling, whether you are (a) taking an undergraduate class and figuring out whether psychotherapy might be a profession for you; (b) taking graduate courses in psychotherapy and ethics; or (c) practicing psychotherapy and exploring ways to become more ethical and or more fulfilled.

A Quick Note on Terminology

Pardon this interruption but we think it is important that we have a common understanding of some terminology. When people write about morals and ethics in philosophy, mental health, medicine, and other fields, they define the words "moral" and "ethical" in a myriad of ways. Some authors use the two terms synonymously; others give them very specific and different meanings. Both terms refer to judgments of right and wrong behavior and the justifications we make for those judgments. In this book we will use the term "ethics" when we are referring to professional behaviors and judgments, and "morals" when we are referring to a wider range of behaviors and judgments including those in personal relationships.

The term *positive ethics* (Handelsman, Knapp, & Gottlieb, 2002; in press) may be a brand new term to you. It refers to the study of ethics as more than a series of rules you must follow to avoid punishment. Behaving ethically by following rules to avoid punishment has been termed *remedial ethics* (Knapp & VandeCreek, 2006). We are all for avoiding punishment, but behaving ethically is not just a matter of following rules – although your professional career might go better when you do. We also believe that professionals are motivated to do good work and actualize their highest moral and ethical selves. It is these higher levels of motivation and behavior that constitute *positive ethics*. We don't think you have to be perfect, but we think focusing on positive themes is more effective, more professionally sustaining, and more fun than focusing on rules and what we shouldn't do.

Mental health professionals use a variety of terms to describe what they do – the two major terms being *psychotherapy* and *counseling*. In the interest of clarity and brevity, we will use the terms counseling, psychotherapy, and therapy interchangeably.

Ethical Acculturation

Behaving ethically and growing toward ethical excellence are complex processes which involve adapting to a new culture – the culture of psychotherapy. This adaptation, which we call *ethical acculturation* (Handelsman, Gottlieb, & Knapp, 2005), involves awareness and action on two major fronts at the same time. The first front is *you*. Who are you, morally and ethically? What is your sense of right and wrong professional behavior? Who have you been throughout your life, in the many types of relationships of which you have been a part? The second front is the *profession of psychotherapy*. The profession of psychotherapy has its own culture, including ethical traditions, values, rules, rituals, and language.

As you begin your acculturation into this new culture, one of the key tasks is to explore this question: "How do I integrate the ethical traditions, values, rules – in short, the culture of psychotherapy – with my own moral intuitions, values, and backgrounds?"

This question or task might take you by surprise. You might be thinking that you already have enough of a personal foundation or moral compass to be an ethical practitioner. For example, (a) you are very motivated to listen and to help people; (b) others tell you that you are a nice person; and (c) you have never been convicted of a felony.

These statements may all be true; however, psychotherapy is a complex profession and the therapeutic relationship includes a unique combination of behaviors and factors.

A major premise of this book is that psychotherapy is both very powerful and very fragile. Like a carefully produced chemical compound, psychotherapy has the potential to cause significant impact on people's lives. On the other hand, if not handled in a diligent manner, psychotherapy can cause great damage. Additionally, when impurities – ethical lapses are equivalent to such foreign substances – enter the picture, psychotherapy can become quite harmful. At the least, such impurities can reduce or destroy the effectiveness of psychotherapy.

This book is a step-by-step guide to ethical acculturation that will help you understand yourself, your ethical culture of origin, and what it means to be or become an ethical psychotherapist. By the way, you will not be finished with your ethical acculturation when you've finished reading this book and made your office furniture purchase. Acculturation is a lifelong process because we change over time – as does the culture of psychotherapy.

Developing a Professional Identity

When you travel to countries with different cultures, you need to be aware of their customs, such as how to show respect, how to negotiate prices, how to communicate gratitude, when to make jokes, and when not to. In a similar way, when you travel to the culture of psychotherapy your ordinary moral sense will take you only so far (Kitchener, 2000). As we engage in the process of ethical acculturation, we formulate a *professional identity*. Our professional identities evolve over time, but we can start now to understand some of the core elements of our identities. The benefits of having a well-thought-out and well-articulated professional identity include providing better psychotherapy to our clients, preventing burnout, and experiencing a more fulfilling and productive career.

We believe there is no real difference between our ethical identities and professional identities because ethical issues are at the heart of good therapy practice. Good therapy naturally means good ethics.

A good professional identity includes four components of moral behavior as outlined by James Rest (1986; Rest & Narváez, 1994).

According to Rest, all four components must occur for moral behavior to occur. The first component is *moral sensitivity*. Ethics is relevant not only when there is a dilemma or you are considering a behavior that is clearly wrong. All of our professional behaviors have ethical components. Moral sensitivity is the ability to discern the ethical dimensions in all our professional activities. The second component is *moral decision-making*. Once we understand the ethical components in a situation, how do we think about these to make our best choices? To be good at moral decision-making means to know a lot about ourselves, ethics, and the profession. In addition, however, good moral decision-making involves a set of reasoning skills that we develop through practice (see chapter 4). The third component is *moral motivation* which refers to the process of identifying our values. Some of them might be in conflict when faced with an ethical decision. Many beginning therapists are surprised to learn that the motivation to help people, while necessary, is not sufficient to be an ethically excellent therapist. Finally, the component of *moral follow-through* refers to acting on our moral beliefs when there are both internal and external factors that may influence us to not act morally.

When you look at these four components, you may be tempted to assume that you already have all these qualities in abundance. You see yourself as sensitive to moral issues, as a moral decision-maker, as one who recognizes competing values or conflicts of interest, and as one who has the internal fortitude to do what is right. You display these qualities regularly in your day-to-day life. However, consider the following two points: (a) even if you possess these qualities now and display them by your choices, you can always develop them more as you engage in the lifelong process of ethical acculturation; (b) once again, we remind you that psychotherapy is different from all other professions and relationships.

On the other hand, you may look at the four components and come to the conclusion that you have none or just a few of these qualities. You may be thinking that becoming (or staying) a therapist is hopeless. We urge you to reserve judgment. It's only the introduction!

Professional Balancing Acts

Our students tell us that becoming a psychotherapist is very enjoyable and rewarding. However, they also tell us of the numerous balancing acts and frustrations that are involved. Each of these balancing acts has important implications for our ethical behavior. The experiences of our young psychotherapist/comedian at the beginning of this chapter highlight the major balancing act inherent in ethical acculturation – between the personal and professional. When we become a professional, or simply start the process, many of our relationships change. For example, your friends might expect to get expert knowledge from you and you just want to be their friend like before! At some point, you might start to think, "Am I moving from giving advice, as any friend would, to giving professional opinions?"

Another sense in which the personal and professional need to be balanced is within our therapy relationships. Our students say things like, "You tell me to use my personality as part of treatment and yet you also say to be professional in the relationship and not just go by my personal experience." Indeed, helping people is much more than common sense or relying on your own experience. At the same time, without understanding your own tendencies, habits, and perceptions as well as using your personality, psychotherapy becomes merely a mechanical process.

The notion of technical knowledge and skill leads us to another balancing act: between humility and competence. Psychotherapists need to know an amazing amount of information about human behavior and develop much skill in applying that knowledge. At the same time, psychotherapists need to know that they cannot help everybody and they will never know everything. Thus, they need to cultivate the virtue of humility and appreciate the limits of their competence – which is determined by their levels of knowledge and skills. The extremes of this balance – feeling like you know everything or feeling like you know nothing – can lead to ethical infractions and burnout.

As a student or practitioner exploring ethical issues, you will face yet another balancing act: between being certain and embracing ambiguity. As you initially study the ethics codes of your discipline, you will find that the codes often read like a long list of "don'ts" that should be followed blindly. Upon closer inspection, however, you will find that most of the rules are not that definite. They are often difficult to implement in simple ways. The ethical principles and guidelines even contradict each other at times. How are we supposed to behave ethically when the rules are neither clear nor absolute? Answering this question takes careful study, long practice, and an open mind. We urge you to become familiar with the ethics codes of your profession, and perhaps of a few related professions. You can find links to over 100 codes or sets of guidelines at kspope.com/ethcodes/index.php.

Another balance that has important ethical implications is between responsibility and respect. "They tell me I am responsible for how therapy goes," new therapists might say, "and yet they tell me that the client is in control." As psychotherapists, we must be responsible for the methods we use to help our clients, but we must also recognize that clients retain the ultimate responsibility for their own lives. Not appreciating this fact might lead us to blur the boundaries of the psychotherapeutic relationship as we take too much responsibility for clients' lives, or push clients into unwise or premature choices. At the same time, the spheres of responsibility are not always that clearly defined. Many of the ethical issues we explore later in the book will revolve around this issue.

We've mentioned the term *boundaries;* one of the most important balancing acts that we as therapists need to master is between the intimacy involved in psychotherapy and the boundaries of that intimacy. Put another way: The intimacy involved in therapy exists in a very restricted range. For example, clients disclose many personal details in the relationship but therapists typically do not. Another quality of therapeutic intimacy is that it should never be transferred into a romantic or sexual relationship, a business relationship, or even a close friendship. Making sure to respect the boundaries of the therapy relationship is a key to making therapy effective. Thus, ethical decisions about boundaries are not only everyday decisions but every-minute decisions.

A broader balancing act is between our psychotherapeutic worldview and alternative worldviews. Psychotherapy is a western invention and includes values and traditions that seem to make more sense in western cultures. For example, many of the western psychotherapeutic approaches stress or value individuality and independence. Other worldviews value interdependence and seeking the best for the community.

At this point, you might be tempted to throw up your hands and say one of two following statements, "I didn't sign up for all these balancing acts. I just want to help people," or, "OK, this is all interesting but I don't have the slightest clue how to maneuver ethically through all of these issues." If this describes you, take a deep breath and let it out slowly. Relax a little. We wrote this book with you in mind. We want to help you successfully acculturate to the world of psychotherapy.

How We Will Help You in the Process of Ethical Acculturation

The three As of our approach to acculturation are:

- Activity
- Awareness
- Actualization

Activity

We don't know you. We don't know the courses you have taken. We don't know the discipline that you are in. What we do know is that we want to help you develop the skill of reflecting upon yourself and your profession in systematic, integrative, and fulfilling ways. Although we are going to focus on universal ethical issues that all psychotherapists face, your professional identity is yours alone. It comprises your thoughts, values, virtues, skills, attitudes, and character. We invite you to be partners with us in actively exploring your identity. Indeed, the core of your learning experience will be your reactions to what we have written. To this end, we have provided three types of activities throughout the book.

The first type of activity is titled "Journal Entries." This activity offers the most formal way to explore and take more responsibility for your learning from this book. With this activity we encourage you to keep a journal where you record your reactions to the reading. You can keep your journal in a hard-copy notebook or a computer file. You might even want to audiotape some entries and transcribe them later. We will make some suggestions for journal entries, but we encourage you to be willing to write down reactions and thoughts about what you read.

The second type of activity we call "Food for Thought." These are opportunities for you to sit back and reflect upon what you're reading and how you relate to it. The third type of activity we call "Red Flag" and "Green Flag" stories which we will introduce in chapter 4. The concept of red flags indicates ethical pitfalls and the concept of green flags indicates ethical excellence. The flag stories contain specific examples of behaviors and attitudes that you can think about, react to, and expand upon.

If you are reading this book for a class, your professor may ask you to do some additional entries or exercises, or ask you to share your work as part of a class discussion. The purpose of every activity is to facilitate your ethical acculturation – to explore yourself, the culture of psychotherapy, and/or the relationship between the two. As you respond to our prompts, remember that there are very few clearly right or wrong answers; we've left most of the questions open-ended to facilitate your exploration.

You probably won't need to do each activity at one sitting. We encourage you to take your time and reflect. Also, you probably won't need to answer every subquestion in every activity. However, we believe the more you do, the more you will benefit from this book. Think of these activities as similar to physical exercises. You need to develop your ethical muscles and these exercises will give you a good workout!

Awareness

We ask you to keep an open mind and to continue expanding your awareness. For example, in our activities we sometimes ask you to take different perspectives. We will ask you to respond as a therapist, but we will also ask you to put yourself in the position of a client, a colleague, or a member of an ethics committee that has to judge whether a particular behavior was ethical or not. These perspectives will help you understand the complexity and uniqueness of psychotherapy.

Most of our suggestions will be worded in such a way as to apply primarily to beginning therapists. However, we think practicing psychotherapists would do well to revisit this book on a regular basis. If you are an experienced therapist, you can easily adapt the activities by thinking about the next stage of your career as a renewal or re-entry into a changing professional culture. But do not modify the activities too much! There is much to be gained from moving back a few steps and casting fresh eyes upon ground that we believe we have already covered.

Food for Thought: *Personal and Professional Relationships*

Here is your first activity: Remember the psychotherapist at the comedy club and all of the family and friends with new expectations? We want to give you some time to think about some of the relationships in your own life that have changed because of your entry into this new profession.

Part 1   Think of some of the personal relationships you are in. For example, you might be a best friend, a child in relation to your parents, a sibling, etc. How have these relationships changed since entering school or since beginning your practice?

Part 2   Now think about the new types of professional relationships you are in because you have begun your studies or practice. For example, you might be a classmate, a practicum student, a psychotherapist, a colleague of other psychotherapists, etc. What makes these professional relationships professional? What makes them different from personal relationships? What qualities or skills do you think you will want to have in place to make the relationships work?

Actualization

One way to think about developing an ethical identity is that it's a way of actualizing your vision of what it means to be a professional. We want to emphasize that developing your ethical muscles can be a positive and personal venture rather than an alienating attempt to follow a disembodied set of rules (Handelsman, Knapp, & Gottlieb, in press). For example, it is unethical for psychotherapists to accept expensive gifts from clients. Many new therapists see this prohibition as an intrusion into the therapeutic relationship and an unnecessary constraint on their behavior. A more positive perspective is to see the acceptance of expensive gifts as outside the boundaries of psychotherapy; it is one of those impurities that might dilute or even destroy the therapeutic relationship. Accepting expensive gifts runs a high risk of compromising our objectivity and promoting a conflict of interest. These work against our desire to produce beneficial therapeutic outcomes and to act in clients' best interests. Thus, not accepting expensive gifts is an expression of our concern for clients and a way to make sure that we provide what we promised to clients.

Journal Entry: *Adjectives*

Take some time to write in your journal: Think about a time in the future when you will have been a psychotherapist for several years and have developed a reputation. What *four adjectives* would you like your *clients* to use when they describe you as a professional? What four adjectives would you like your *colleagues* to use to describe you as a professional? Why have you chosen these adjectives? What do they reflect about you?

What This Book Is Not

We have written this book to be different from other ethics books, some of which you may be using along with this one. The first difference it that this book is not discipline-specific. We have written it for all who are or will be performing psychotherapy, including counselors, marriage and family therapists, psychiatrists, psychologists, social workers and others. Thus, we will not provide a comprehensive guide to every ethical situation covered by other discipline-specific ethics books.

The second difference is that this book is not a set of rules to follow in every situation. We will provide some answers about what to do in some situations (like the previous example with the expensive gift), but we are more interested in helping you develop your ability to (a) recognize ethical issues because you are more sensitized to them; (b) think about ethical issues from a knowledgeable position; (c) integrate what you read in the ethics codes with who you are as a person and professional; and (d) develop the character strengths to act in concert with your convictions. If we achieve these goals, you will be more likely to follow your ethics codes now and as they evolve in the future.

Journal Entry: *Chapter Reflections*

Here is your second journal entry. We have posed some questions to help you reflect on this chapter.

- How did you react to this first chapter?
- What surprised you about what we said?
- What parts of the chapter seemed to make the most sense and what parts were counterintuitive?
- Did you find yourself getting defensive at anything we said? What?
- What are you most looking forward to about this book? What are you least looking forward to?

This is a journal entry that you can repeat at the end of *every* chapter!

Food for Thought: *What Would You Do?*

First scenario: In an ethics class of Sharon's, a scenario came up in discussion about an armored truck having an accident right outside the building and money spilling out into the street. One of the students said, "I'd pick up as much as I could! The money doesn't belong to anyone." Another student said, "But it doesn't belong to you." A third student said, "Wow, I don't know what I would do. I guess maybe it would depend on whether my family was struggling financially."

- What are your reactions to these statements?
- What would you do in that situation, and why?

Now change the scenario a bit. Suppose the accident happened right outside your psychotherapy office and your client and colleagues are watching the same scene.

- What would you do?
- Would your response be the same as it was in the previous scene? Why or why not?

Notice the kinds of arguments you made. Your justifications for your courses of action are reflections of your ethical and moral background, your values, and your sense of what it means to be a professional.

Coming Attractions

In the next two chapters we will ask you to think more about your background and how it might prepare you for your professional roles. In chapter 3, we will discuss in more detail the process of acculturation and how to develop your professional identity. Readers who want a broad overview before getting into specifics may want to read chapter 3 first.

Part I

Taking Stock

1

Basics of Awareness
Knowing Yourself

We open this chapter with a story from Mitch:

> When I reached middle age (early, early, middle age), we got a treadmill to get some exercise. I was very anxious to get started, so I just turned the machine on, got the tread revolving, and started walking. On the model we bought, there are about twenty different built-in programs that simulate everything from a power walk to a climb up a hill at heart-pumping speed. There are hundreds of different settings, none of which I've used in ten years!

As you are reading this scenario you might be thinking, "Wow Mitch, what a waste. You are really missing out on some good exercise." And you are right! By Mitch not familiarizing himself with the basic machinery – not reading the instructions nor doing some systematic assessment – he's missing out on a high level of effectiveness even though he gets an adequate amount of exercise. Or you might be thinking, "No big deal Mitch; you're getting enough exercise. Listen, there's no need to bother with all the bells and whistles." You might be right on this view too. For a home treadmill, this may be a perfectly fine way to go. After all, it's Mitch's money; he can do with it as he pleases. He's not influencing anybody else.

But the scenario and our responses change when we're talking about a professional activity with potentially huge impacts – positive or negative – on other people. This is when positive ethics come into play. When we involve positive ethics, we are obligated to do more than the minimum. We need to move beyond the ethical floor (staying out of trouble) and shoot for the ethical ceiling (excellent and exemplary professional practice) (Handelsman, Knapp, & Gottlieb, 2002; Knapp & VandeCreek, 2006).

Think about your graduate school applications: Did you say you wanted to be adequate, to help people *a little*, to be only as good a therapist as you need to avoid being complained about? Similar to the treadmill scenario, merely doing some quick walking on the treadmill and not falling off is not reaping the benefits of a well equipped machine! To shoot for the ethical ceiling means more than just following rules and staying out of trouble. When you do good work and stay motivated, you do so in a personal and professional context that makes sense and resonates with both your head and heart. Corey, Corey, and Callanan (2007) state that a major piece of psychotherapy is the person part of the therapist which includes the psychotherapist's values, needs, and personal motivations.

We wholeheartedly agree. We want help you gain a solid working knowledge of your own ethical origins, a clear understanding of how positive ethics is possible, and an appreciation for the relationship between ethics and excellent therapeutic practice.

At this point you might be thinking, "OK, already, you've convinced me. Let's get on with it. Just show me the ethics! I'll follow the rules. Just let me get started!" To this we say, "Hold on!" We encourage you to explore who you are morally and ethically as well as to take some time to learn about the "treadmill" – learn about the psychotherapy culture. Here we dedicate some time to explore the pre-existing workout programs – explore your personal morals and values that you are bringing into your new profession. And then we can examine how you might modify your workout – assess the match or mismatch between the profession's culture and your personal ethics, values, and morals.

We want you to achieve the high goals you have for your work by using every bit of your professional knowledge and putting your virtuous character to work. That's why in this chapter we focus on you. We're not going to talk (yet) about rules to follow. Rather, we're going to ask you to look at your feelings, motivations, values, virtues, and moral courage. These elements contribute to your personal and professional knowledge, skills, and attitudes necessary in order to do more than follow the rules. In other words, we want you to develop a comprehensive and coherent ethical identity as a professional.

For us, positive ethics includes codes and rules but moves beyond them to explore the moral dimensions of the profession. This exploration is accomplished through the lenses of values, virtues, self-care, ethical decision-making, sensitivity, valuing the moral foundations of ethics codes, and encouraging positive behaviors (Kuther, 2003). The foundation of positive ethics begins with understanding yourself in the context of the profession. So let's get started on our exploration.

Food for Thought: *Feelings, Nothing More Than Feelings*

How are you feeling about becoming (being) a psychotherapist? Scared? Excited? Intimidated? Impatient? Fulfilled? Picture yourself in therapy sessions with a variety of different kinds of clients (e.g., tall, short, female, male, Native American, White, Black, Asian, Hispanic, heterosexual, homosexual, homeless, rich, able-bodied, wheelchair-bound, motivated, unmotivated, clean, dirty, attractive, unattractive, old, young, genteel, foul-mouthed, thin, obese, urban, rural, liberal, conservative, communist, Christian, Jewish, Muslim, Hindu, orthodox, atheist, truck-driver, rock star, psychotherapist). Now picture the "perfect" client and list all the feelings you have, especially as you anticipate being in a session with this person. Next, picture your least favorite client and list all the feelings you might have as you anticipate seeing this person. Our emotions are a critical part of our experience with clients. They inform us about our prejudices, biases, preferences, and values.

From reading your other textbooks, or from what you have heard from your colleagues, classmates, and professors, you might be feeling overwhelmed. You might have said something like this to yourself: "There's too much; I don't know how to handle it. I hear people talking about confidentiality, reporting child abuse, boundaries, multiple relationships – how do I keep all this straight!" If this is the case, we draw upon the treadmill analogy and say, "It seems intimidating now because you haven't even read the instructions yet!" When you see the flashing lights on the treadmill that read, "Choose your program," you feel helpless only because you haven't prepared yourself with information to make a choice.

The opposite reaction is to be *under*whelmed as you anticipate being a psychotherapist or meeting with your current clients. You might be asking yourself, "Why are ethics such a big deal? It seems like there are so many rules – Don't do this and don't do that! What's wrong with 'If it feels good, do it'? I am a nice person and I care about clients – isn't that enough?" You may be reacting like Mitch did when he first stepped on the treadmill: "Just show me how to make that thing move, and I'll take it from there. I don't need to bother with the preliminaries and the extras." You might be a bit impatient and want to move on a little more quickly than is wise.

Here's our suggestion: Relax a little, no matter what you are thinking and feeling about your professional journey. We want you to take one step at a time and make an investment in the material of this chapter. It will pay off, both for you and your clients.

Motivations

As a part of your ethical identity, your motivations for being a psychotherapist are analogous to the fuel or energy that propels the new treadmill. Unlike simple machines, however, the sources of energy – your motivations – are many and varied. When we review the statements of interest written by prospective students, we always come across a number of noble motivations: "I want to help people as a way to change the world by relieving the suffering of individuals." Often, these noble motivations seem to match up well with personal characteristics and stated experiences of students: "I was always the one whom my friends confided in. I guess that means I'm a good listener," or, "My friends typically look to me for guidance. If they have a problem, I'm the one they contact," or, "I like to help people and seem to be pretty good at it. My friends tell me I am a natural. I think this makes me a good match for being a therapist."

Such noble motivations and basic skills are important, but they are merely the tip of the iceberg. There are thousands of other motivations which can and typically do run the gamut from the highest motives to change the world to very personal and individual ones. Sometimes we are aware of other motives, although we refrain from listing them on graduate school applications because they don't seem relevant or because we're a little ashamed of them. For example, most of us want and need to earn money to make a living. We also want to be in a profession that enjoys some prestige. Other times our motives are hidden, even from us. We might be motivated by power, personal prestige, or other personal drives. Uncovering the personal needs that drive our motivations for becoming a psychotherapist is important (Bashe, Anderson, Handelsman, & Klevansky, 2007). Here's an example of why it's important to understand the personal needs. This is from Sharon:

> I realized during my internship year that one of my motivations to become a psychotherapist grew out of a subconscious drive to make sense of my own family dynamics. This realization came to light while working with an estranged couple. I saw the husband as not caring and aloof and the wife as emotionally neglected and fragile. I felt good about my work with this couple until my supervisor viewed a session on tape. At one point she stopped the tape and pointed out how I had really aligned myself with the wife and joined her in verbally mistreating her husband. My first response was shock. My next response was "Ouch!" My professional ego had been pinched! My subconscious need to "fix" a family-of-origin relationship compromised my ability to connect with the husband of this couple. I wasn't listening well and I was not being helpful to my clients. In this case, my purely personal motivation inhibited my professional motivation. (We'll mention this story again in chapter 8 on supervision.)

Some personal motives, however, are appropriate – in the right amount – to merge with professional ones. Think of nitroglycerine: In small doses, it can keep people alive. In larger doses, it can blow people up. Small doses of some personal motivations, balanced with professional motivations and sensitivity, will work well together. For example, a little psychological voyeurism (wanting to hear about other people's private lives) might be a good thing when combined with compassion, respect, helping, and objectivity. The voyeurism might keep you interested! Another example is your financial and power motives. These two motives, used appropriately, allow you to do what you do and to achieve your larger goals of helping and service.

The bottom line: Psychotherapy is a profession, which means you don't just get to do what you want to do. Your *primary* motivations need to be professional and moral (Rest, 1983, 1994; Kitchener, 2000), even though your personal motivations play a role.

Journal Entry: *Motivations*

In this activity we'll be asking you to dig deep and share some of the most personal and private elements of your professional identity. Therefore, we suggest that you complete at least the first two parts of this entry in a very private place where you can be honest with yourself.

Part 1   Answer the following questions as truthfully as you can: Why do (or did) you want to be a psychotherapist? When you think back (or forward) to completing your application for graduate school, what were your top three reasons for applying? What personal needs are getting met by being or becoming a psychotherapist?

   Be inclusive in your list of motivations. Certainly include the noble motivations, the ones you discussed on your applications (e.g., helping people live better lives). But also include the base motivations, the more "human" and personal ones (e.g., a sense of power, having an office rather than a cubicle, comfortable chairs, prestige, the enjoyment of being needed, hearing stories of others, or wanting to save others from the kind of family you had). Go beyond what you know and speculate about some motivations that you *might* have even if you are not in touch with them at the moment. Remember Sharon's story? If she had done this exercise during her training before internship, she might have uncovered the hidden need to understand family dynamics and been less likely to align herself with only one part of the couple.

Part 2   After you have generated as complete a list of motivations as you can, think about how central each motivation is or might be. Rate each motivation on a scale from 1 to 5, with 1 being "just a little important," and 5 being "absolutely critical to my being a therapist." One way to make these judgments is to ask yourself how you would feel about being a therapist if a particular motivation were not satisfied. For example, if "having a big office with nice furniture" is one of your motivations, what would it do to your desire to be a therapist if we told you (just for the sake of argument) that that motivation would definitely not be satisfied during your career?

Part 3   Think about your *second choice* of a career. What would you be doing or going to school for if not for becoming a psychotherapist? This second-choice career could be something totally apart from the mental health fields or it could be something related, like psychology research. Once you have picked a second-choice career, list the motivations that you have or would have for that career. Repeat the ratings that you did in Part 2 for this new list of motivations. What are the similarities and differences between the motivations and their importance for the two careers?

Food for Thought: *Professional Motivation*

Think about a professional you've seen – a therapist, accountant, nurse, etc. As you picture yourself listening to and taking their advice, think about *their* motives. What might their central and peripheral motivations be? Which are acceptable to you, which are not? Which ones might get in the way of their providing useful services to you? Which might be unacceptable and irrelevant to you at the same time?

Think about a time when you've worked with a professional whose motives you questioned, if only to yourself. What made you wonder about them? Words? Behaviors? Subtle cues?

Values

Another element of your professional identity is your values. What's important to you? What would the world look like if things were perfect? Values overlap with motivations to a substantial degree; we are often driven to actualize our values. However, sometimes our motives conflict with our values, or our values conflict with each other. For example, you think having a fuel-efficient (and expensive) automobile is desirable but your motivation to help people without access to mental health care keeps you working at the local mental health center for a low salary.

Like your motivations, some of your values are purely personal, some purely professional, and some a combination. Some of your personal values might be: "I believe it's important to make money. I believe it's important to provide for my family. Personal growth is important." We can talk about professional values in regard to what you think is important for your profession – and for you as a professional – to be, do, or accomplish. One of your professional values might be "I think it's important to help other people grow." Some of the personal and professional values will be moral values which have to do with your relationships to other people: helping them, respecting them, and fulfilling duties. The intersection of your moral and professional values is where your sense of professional ethics comes from. We hope you can actualize most of your professional and personal values at least over the course of a career, if not every hour of every day.

Also like motives, values can range from noble to base. Some of your values probably revolve around the human condition and the desire to see people thrive and grow. Obviously, these values match well with many of the goals of psychotherapy and overlap with your desire to be a therapist. Some of your values, however, may revolve around financial, social, and personal success and stability. Being a successful psychotherapist is clearly a way to actualize these values. Of course, our values are complex and the likelihood of dealing with conflicting values is very high.

Journal Entry: *Values, Nothing More than Values*

Similar to the list of motivations you created for being a therapist, generate a list of your values. Each value on your list can start this way: "I think it's important ..." After you've done that, make them into a hierarchy. Which ones are most important? Which ones are least important? Which ones would you consider central to your role as a psychotherapist? Which ones would be especially important in terms of your professional ethics?

Why create these lists of motivations and values? First, you need to be aware of as many of your motivations as possible because not all of them will be satisfied at any given time. For example, some psychotherapy clients change very little or not at all. The value you attach to helping may not be fully actualized when you don't see a client improving. At times like these, you need to be aware of *all* your motives for being a psychotherapist.

Second, as we mentioned before, some values will often conflict with each other. Indeed, one way to assess and better understand our values is to explore the choices we make when values and motives conflict (Abeles, 1980).

Third, it's important to know the difference between values and the expression or implementation of values. Sometimes it will appear that the values you hold will conflict with those of the psychotherapy profession when the problem is really one of expression. We may value compassion, but we can't show our compassion with clients in the same way we do with friends (hugging, lending money, sharing our problems, etc.).

Fourth, sometimes your values and the values of psychotherapy will actually be in conflict. We'll be getting to that in chapter 3.

Food for Thought: *Exploring Personal Motivations and Values*

You see a client who is a little anxious about his local acting job. The client tells you wonderful, funny stories about his life and his family. You are fascinated, at times spellbound, by the client's dramatic way of speaking. He is a pleasure to work with because he is professionally rewarding – he's making progress in therapy – and personally engaging. Several months later, the client appears on a local news program telling those same stories as part of his one-man show. Within a few months your former client is a "hit" on Broadway. You see him now on national talk shows; he even mentions his "shrink" in some of his interviews. You feel the urge to brag to your friends that *you're* the "shrink" and that you helped him get where he is today.

Explore your motivations: Why do you want to tell others? To feel powerful or important? To impress your friends? To become, perhaps, a bit of a celebrity yourself? Under what values are you operating? See if the motivations and values you list here are similar to what you listed in your last two journal entries.

Virtues and Moral Courage

You may feel like you've done all you need to do to meet the ethical requirements of psychotherapy and we could stop here, with motivations and values. But we've only gone through part of the instruction manual of our ethics treadmill. Ethics is not just about accepting and then conforming your behavior to the rules. An effective and rewarding professional identity includes developing moral habits that are so ingrained they become personality characteristics.

In addition to considering what you should do and not do, excellent ethical practice requires that we spend some quality time considering *whom you should be* as a professional. In other words, let's talk about *virtues* (Jordan & Meara, 1990; Meara, Schmidt, & Day, 1996; Peterson & Seligman, 2004). Peterson and Seligman (2004) have outlined six basic virtues along with associated character strengths, outlined below:

I   Wisdom and knowledge
  • Creativity
  • Curiosity
  • Open-mindedness
  • Love of learning
  • Perspective
II Courage
  • Bravery
  • Persistence
  • Integrity
  • Vitality
III Humanity
  • Love
  • Kindness
  • Social intelligence
IV Justice
  • Citizenship
  • Fairness
  • Leadership
V   Temperance
  • Forgiveness
  • Humility
  • Prudence
  • Self-regulation
VI Transcendence
  • Appreciation of beauty and excellence
  • Gratitude
  • Hope
  • Humor
  • Spirituality

For our purposes, we can consider all of them virtues. Some of the virtues that good psychotherapists might cultivate include integrity, prudence, humility, compassion, respectfulness, and truthfulness.

It could be argued that it is unnecessary to think in terms of virtues. You might be tempted to think: "If I follow the rule to tell the truth, that's good enough! Isn't it?" In most cases, the answer is probably yes. But which of the following phrases fits better with your conception of whom you'd like to be as a psychotherapist?

- I told the truth because it was a rule I needed to follow and I didn't want to get into trouble.
- I told the truth because I am a truthful professional and to not tell the truth would have resulted in internal discord.

Cultivating virtues, in addition to following the rules, gives us a chance to feel more connected to our profession and to create a coherent identity.

Too much or too little of a virtue can be problematic. For example, too little compassion leads to indifference and too much compassion may lead to problems like taking too much responsibility for clients or enabling their self-defeating behaviors. Here's another example: Too little humility leads to arrogance and too much humility can lead to self-debasement and timidity.

It is useful to think about cultivating an optimal amount of each of our virtues. Additionally, virtues do not exist in isolation; they should exist in an optimal combination. Consider the virtue of truthfulness. Sometimes we don't tell a client the entire truth. For instance, we may not tell one client in the marriage what the other has said about them in a private therapy session. Our virtue of truthfulness needs to be tempered by considerations based on virtues such as respectfulness (the spouse shared impressions in private and expects his or her privacy to be respected) and prudence (sharing the information at this time in therapy may cause more harm than good).

The virtues of *integrity* and *prudence* may be central virtues. You can think of integrity as the state of having all the other virtues in proper proportions and balance, and prudence as the practical wisdom to decide how to express those virtues in the widest possible variety of situations.

Virtues, like motives and values, can be separated into personal and professional, with a subset of moral virtues. Once again, we'd like you to consider the moral virtues that you wish to cultivate in your professional activities.

Food for Thought: *Virtues*

Part 1 In your journal, create a list of three virtues that you express, at least some of the time, in your life. For each of these virtues, answer this question: When you are not being perfectly virtuous, what end do you flip to? For example, if you consider yourself a compassionate person, when you are not perfectly compassionate, do you feel too much (get in a person's way by making a decision for them) or too little (neglect to give a person the basic support and guidance needed)?

Part 2 Think about several kinds of situations you face in your life and see if there are variations in your expression of virtues. For example, if you thought of truthfulness, how does the amount of truthfulness change depending upon whom you are dealing with, the type of situation, the kinds of behavior called for, and other considerations? Think, for example, about somebody you are very close to, somebody with whom you have a professional relationship, and somebody who is merely an acquaintance. Think about a work situation, a personal situation, and/or a family situation.

Part 3
- What would your friends consider your greatest virtue? Your weakest?
- What do you hope your clients will or do say about you?
- What do you hope your colleagues will or do say about you?
- What new virtue will you most want to develop in your role as a psychotherapist?
- What is your plan for how you might develop this virtue?

One potential danger in thinking about your own virtues is believing that, because you have desirable personality traits, you are immune from unethical behavior. Most psychotherapists, and those training to become psychotherapists, know right from wrong. It is a myth that most psychotherapists who engage in unethical or unprofessional behavior are sociopaths with no consciences and no virtues. In reality, every professional is capable of unethical conduct.

So, why do good psychotherapists who know what is right sometimes choose to do what's wrong? This question is complex – in a sense, this entire book is an attempt to explore the answers to this question. Let's look at one possible reason that relates to moral motivation and moral follow-through: Sometimes we know what the right thing to do is, but we also know that some of the outcomes of the right action will result in difficulties or hardships for us. Consider these examples:

- A client of yours has been doing pretty well in therapy. One day he tells you that he has abused his child. You know that you are required to report the abuse to the local Social Service agency and you could lose your license to practice if you don't report. You also know or assume that if you do report your client he will stop treatment and the possibility of further improvement (as well as future payment) is taken away.

- A friend of yours, a fellow psychotherapy student, is pressed for time and so writes up an assessment report on a client without doing all the necessary tests. In fact, he makes up some of the scores for an intelligence test. When you confront him about his behavior, he tells you that he knows the client well enough to estimate the scores and no harm will be done. He goes on to tell you that if he doesn't turn in his report he could get fired from the clinic and maybe kicked out of the training program. He's been your loyal friend since the first day of grad school and has done you some favors during stressful times. You know he has the potential to be a fine therapist. He asks you to do him this one teensy little favor and not turn him in for his dishonesty.

- You notice that the mental health center at which you are working has overbilled a state agency for the treatment of several indigent patients. You inform your supervisor, expecting her immediately to thank you for telling her so that she can let her superiors know that they need to reimburse the state. Instead, she tells you that many patients (who are not part of the state program) do not pay their bills and without the money from the state the center might have to go out of business. "If we didn't get that money some other center would, and we need it more." She makes it clear that good employees of the center would not make such a fuss and that employees who do don't remain employees for long.

In each of these situations, you face the possibility of unpleasant consequences for doing the right thing. The ability to do the right thing in these types of situations is called *moral courage*. When we face an ethical problem and need to implement a difficult decision, it is our moral courage – also called "moral character" (Rest, 1983, 1994) or "resoluteness" (Betan & Stanton, 1999) – that carries us through to complete our ethical course of action. In short, we can define moral courage as the demonstration of any of our moral virtues or values in the face of personal distress or discomfort.

Ethics Autobiography – Part 1

Now that you've identified the motivations, values, and virtues that may drive much of your professional behavior, how do you put these together to make decisions about right and wrong, ethical and unethical? How do you actualize your vision of what it means to be an ethical professional? How have you learned, so far in your life, about right and wrong professional behavior? We are not asking these as prescriptive questions – we're not asking how you *should* make those decisions. We are asking the questions about how you think *right now* about such issues, and how you may have developed your intuitive notions of professional ethics.

Earlier, Sharon shared her story of working with a couple, at least in part, in such a way so as to "fix" some of her own unconscious family dynamics. Clearly, this is wrong, because we are not there to help solve our personal problems. But how do we know when an action or behavior is unethical? How do we make those decisions? In this section, we want you to explore where you are (and have been) morally, how you know when professional behaviors are right or wrong.

The personal/professional *ethics autobiography* is described in a previous work by us with two of our colleagues (Bashe et al., 2007). We have used this activity over the years as we teach undergraduate and graduate ethics courses. The main purpose of our version of an ethics autobiography is to encourage self-reflection about your personal ethics of origin. This is your existing instruction manual, wiring diagram, and troubleshooting guide for your built-in moral machinery. The more you know about it, the more you can use it to help develop your professional ethical muscles!

We'll introduce the second part of the ethics autobiography later when we've introduced the basics of the culture of psychotherapy. For now, let's get a sense of who you are, morally.

Journal Entry: *Ethics Autobiography, Part 1*

Put the following on the top of a new page in your journal: name, date, context (meaning graduate school, employment, or wherever you are in your professional journey) and anything else that will help make a connection for you about the time and place for this journal entry.

Next, address the following questions:

1. What motivations, values, and virtues are most important to you, as a person, in your relationships with other people? You might want to refer to some of your previous journal entries.
2. What are the origins of these motivations, values, and virtues? Be inclusive. Don't just write, "I was born with them." Take some time to really think about where you might have learned your values. For example, from family members? Religious figures? What you learned in school? Teachers or professors? Coaches? Bosses?
3. How similar are your motivations, values, and virtues to those of other members of the cultures to which you belong? By culture, we mean any group of people who share some values, traditions, or ideals. Your nationality, religion, gender, geographic area, and sexual orientation are all cultures. You can even think more broadly. Mitch, for example, belongs to the cultures of trumpet players, contact lens wearers, and full professors.
4. What experiences have you had with members of cultures to which you do not belong and their notions of right and wrong?

What feelings did you have about those experiences and about the members of those other cultures?

5. At this stage in your professional journey, what would you consider as examples of right and wrong *professional* behavior?

6. Where does your idea of right and wrong professional behavior come from?

7. How might your motivations, values, and virtues that you wrote about in questions 1–3 influence your decisions about right and wrong professional behavior?

8. As you've answered the preceding questions, what thoughts and feelings are stirred in you? How do your journal entries about motivations and values sound now as you reread them?

What you've written is the *beginning* of a *rough draft* of your autobiography. Your autobiography, like your growth and development as a professional, *will never be finished* because your experiences, thoughts, and perspectives will change over time. So keep this portion of your journal accessible, as you will have occasion to refer back to it, reconceptualize it, and revise it many times.

Basics of Self-care

Earlier in this chapter we made the point that some of your personal motivations and needs – motivations and needs that contribute to your being human – cannot be actualized or acted upon as a therapist. These needs will have to be met elsewhere. Even some of the professional motivations will not be entirely met in the therapy room. To avoid inappropriate needs spilling over into the therapeutic relationship, you need to develop the skills, knowledge, and awareness necessary to get your nontherapeutic needs met so they do not contaminate the therapeutic relationship. We are talking about self-care.

Self-care begins with awareness on two levels. The first level is self-awareness. In the journal entry "Motivations," we asked you, "What personal needs are getting met by being or becoming a psychotherapist?" Take a look back at what you wrote: If you didn't answer this question earlier, take some time to answer it now. If you did answer it, see if anything else occurs to you. Be tenaciously truthful with yourself.

The second level of awareness is to be honest with ourselves about the nature of our professional activities. Clearly there are immense rewards for being a therapist and many find it a truly noble way to make a living. At the same time, psychotherapy is taxing and emotionally draining; authors have used phrases like "significantly stressful" (Cottone & Tarvydas, 2007, p. 123), and "inherently stressful" (Welfel, 2006, p. 58). The scenario looks something like this: We work with clients who are unhappy, ineffective, dissatisfied, angry, anxious, and/or lonely, and who sometimes really want to stay unhappy, ineffective, dissatisfied, angry, anxious, and lonely. Under these conditions, they challenge us to be that person in their lives who brings hope, a point of connection, stability, and caring confrontation. The increments of change we may see during the therapy process are often very small. In addition to this, we may rarely know of the positive endings for clients, which may happen long after termination. Thus, we often do not fully collect on the promise of good feelings after a job well done.

These conditions, plus other factors that may be out of our control (e.g., reimbursement from insurance carriers), constitute a recipe for emotional exhaustion. We need strategies to prevent the harmful effects of these stresses and to help ourselves when we start to feel detached, overwhelmed, and burned out (Jevne & Williams, 1998). We need to be on guard for the telltale signs of such stress, like fleeting hopes that our clients call to cancel their appointments, impatience with our clients, and musing between sessions about going back to school to study geology. You need to be your own best friend and make a strong commitment to take care of yourself. Those who need your help – your clients – won't be asking you if you are getting good rest at night, taking periodic vacations, exercising regularly, or are involved in healthy personal relationships. You need to be checking in on yourself and seeking assistance from colleagues. For now, let's look at stress and how you recharge your batteries.

Food for Thought: *Stress*

1. What is or has been your most stressful work experience?
2. What do (did) you do about that stress?

3. What do (did) you see other people doing?
4. What do (did) you do about stress at school?
5. What could you do to cope better?
6. Choose one coping activity and start doing it now!

Researchers Jane Myers, Thomas Sweeney, and J. Melvin Witmer (2000) describe the concept of *wellness* as "a way of life oriented toward optimal health and well-being in which body, mind and spirit are integrated by the individual to live more fully within the human and natural community" (p. 252). Personal wellness is critical for our own well-being and our professional excellence. Spending time and effort on ourselves is part of our ethical obligation, in addition to the time and effort we spend on behalf of our clients. As Thomas Skovholt, a noted counseling psychologist at the University of Minnesota, states, "Maintaining oneself personally is necessary to function effectively in a professional role. By itself, this idea can help those in the caring fields feel less selfish when meeting the needs of the self" (2001, p. 146). In an important sense, wellness is to stress reduction as positive ethics is to ethics – it allows us to go beyond the minimum and reach a higher level.

Food for Thought: *Specific Wellness Strategies*

As a way to evaluate your self-care, consider the following list of categories. For each category, give yourself a rating of 0–5, with 0 meaning *"no self-care"* and 5 meaning *"good self-care"* in the category.

_____ I encourage myself to feel.
_____ I have my finances in good-to-great shape.
_____ I have a laugh at least once during each day.
_____ I give other people, as well as myself, a compliment most every day.
_____ I have a healthy diet when it comes to food.

_____ I walk and/or get exercise sometime during my day.

_____ I have hobbies or activities that I do only for fun.

_____ I keep my life's priorities front and center and don't let the tyranny of the urgent draw me off course.

_____ I stop and just breathe when my day starts to feel stressful.

_____ I give myself permission to be alone when I need solitary time.

_____ I take time to foster my spiritual or religious self.

_____ I have at least one healthy relationship in my life.

Now go back over your list and see if there are any scores you wish to change. If yes, write an action plan for one of those items. Keep this list handy so that you can retrieve it on a regular basis. We would suggest that you do this activity at least twice a year.

In spite of the inherent stress of psychotherapy, there are ways to stay vibrant in the profession. Skovholt (2001) encourages professionals to seek out those experiences in their personal lives that promote happiness, fervor, energy, and tranquility. Of course, the list you develop to experience these will likely look different from those of your colleagues or classmates. That's fine. The key is to make the list and then implement your list on a regular basis. It is also important to remember that your list will change over the years as you develop as a person and a professional.

Journal Entry: *Staying Vibrant*

Make a list of the experiences, activities, behaviors, and thoughts that provide you with a sense of happiness, fervor, energy, and/or tranquility. *Do not list anything that has to do with your professional activities!* Your list should be a personal one, not a professional one. Once again, we encourage you to be inclusive and to put on your list, even things that provide only a little happiness.

2
Basics of Awareness
Privilege and Social Responsibility

We begin this chapter with a story by Sharon:

> I want to share with you a little of my journey of coming to know
> my privilege (for an extended version of this story, see Anderson &
> Middleton, 2005a), which has been a very important part of my
> own ethical acculturation journey. I share this story to highlight
> several features of the process: First, becoming aware of one's
> point(s) of privilege can be uncomfortable, sometimes even emo-
> tionally and psychologically painful. Second, being willing to have
> what I call "difficult dialogues" with individuals different from
> ourselves about points of privilege, discrimination, and oppression –
> keeping our minds and hearts open as we exchange our percep-
> tions and experiences – is hard work. It's as hard as it is important
> on our continuing attempts at fuller awareness. Third, growing
> awareness in this area is a journey that never ends – it is a process.
> Allowing our inner selves to let down the defenses and see privi-
> lege, oppression, and discrimination in a subjective way (including
> ourselves in the mix) is an important first step in the process.
>
> When I was in graduate school I received an evening phone call
> from a friend who was living and working in the southeastern US.
> My friend, Cella (who at the time described herself as an African
> American woman), was frustrated by an experience she had that
> very day. Standing in a long line waiting to order lunch at a fast
> food establishment, Cella was ignored by the counter person. She
> was ready with her order and had moved up to be the next person
> to state her choices when
>
> "The employee, a White woman, looked right past me and asked this
> person who was right behind me and who just happened to be White,

'May I help you?' I was so mad I could have just, just … I don't know. She just ignored me – like I wasn't even there. The people here are so discriminatory against people of color! I can't wait to be transferred out of here!"

As I spoke with Cella about the event, I remember trying to use words that conveyed support, understanding, and empathy. But I also remember thinking to myself, "Cella, you are too sensitive. No one is that rude. You probably just didn't look like you were ready to order."

As life sometimes works out, I had an opportunity a few years later to see this same scene play out before my very eyes. Val (a Black woman) and I had lunch at a restaurant, during which we had what I called one of our "difficult dialogues" about racism and discrimination. Val wanted me to hear her stories and the stories of others who are seen and treated differently because of their skin color. I wanted to deflect the issues of oppression and discrimination by claiming that White people are treated poorly as well. We finished our conversation with the idea that bringing people together to talk about the issues of privilege and oppression was important. We decided to speak to someone at the establishment about holding lunch meetings at the restaurant. Val was several steps ahead of me as we approached the counter to ask for the manager. The young White lady behind the counter looked right past Val and asked me, "How can I help you?" In that moment the scene that Cella had described to me a few years before came flooding back to my mind. For various reasons, my psychological defenses were down enough to see how my White skin made me visible and how Val's Black skin made her invisible. This was a starting point for my awareness about points of privilege.

Food for Thought: *Hello! I'm Right Here – Why Can't You See Me?*

Think of a time in your life when you were in a meeting or a setting where people around you spoke about you or spoke for you as if you weren't even there. What was the meeting or setting about? Who was there? What is your best guess about what made you "invisible" to every-one around you? How did it feel? What did you want to say to become visible? If you did say something, what was it and did it have an impact? Finally, how far back in time did you need to go to find your example? To when you were a child? Yesterday? This morning?

Before we look at the process of ethical acculturation in the next section of this book, we want to discuss one more level of awareness – social awareness, which includes issues of privilege, discrimination, and social responsibility. We believe these issues form parts of our ethical cultures of origin, our personal values and motivations, and our assumptions about others as individuals or as members of a larger group – parts that are not often recognized as such but are important to consider as we develop our professional identities. The examination of personal points of privilege and discrimination relates to the larger issue of social responsibility – how we implement on a broader scale the personal virtues (e.g., respect, humility, compassion, fairness) and values that we addressed in chapter 1. Being able to see points of privi-lege, discrimination, and oppression – in reference to ourselves and others – can help us actualize our virtues and values, achieve ethical excellence in our personal and professional lives, and avoid harm to our clients.

Privilege

Peggy McIntosh is a research scientist at the Wellesley Centers for Women and a pioneer in the field. McIntosh (1990) used the term "White privilege" when she realized that as a White person she had access and opportunities or advantages that others did not. She described White privilege as that "invisible package of unearned assets" that those of us who have White skin "can count on cashing in each day" without a second thought (p. 13). But White privilege is just one type or point of privilege. Other points include male privilege, able-bodied privilege, economic privilege, and heterosexual privilege. As individuals we have multiple identities (Tatum, 1999). In some ways or contexts we may experience privilege (because we are part of a dominant group) and in others we may experience discrimination or oppression (Lo, 2005). We can experience a type of "mental whiplash, alternating … between disadvantaged and privileged group memberships" (Liddle, 2005, p. 171). We might even have both experiences at the same time in the same place.

Without some prompting, we might be unaware of, or remain oblivious to, our invisible package of privilege and discrimination. This state of unawareness may be an outcome of learning. McIntosh states it this way: "As a White person, I realized I had been taught about racism as something that puts others at a disadvantage, but had been taught not to see one of its corollary aspects, White privilege, which puts me at an advantage" (p. 31). Dr McIntosh is not alone in this experience. In our own individual or personal context or environment, we are typically not taught to notice those ways we have "advantages"; we really just come to see them as the expected.

In our formal training as psychotherapists we get exposed to many multicultural issues and competencies; however, we might not be encouraged or taught to see our own points of privilege – our unearned assets. When we don't see our own privilege we will likely find it difficult to see discrimination against, and possible oppression of, others (Anderson & Middleton, 2005b; Loomis, 2005; Megivern, 2005), including clients and colleagues.

Food for Thought: *Your Own Invisible Knapsack of Privilege*

Sometimes it is hard to think of ourselves as having advantages in life or as living with unearned assets that provide us opportunities that others do not have. We'd like to give you an opportunity to explore what might be in your own "knapsack of privilege" by assessing how your experience matches these statements. The more you respond in the affirmative the more likely you are to have one or more points of privilege (male privilege, able-bodied privilege, economic privilege, heterosexual privilege, religious privilege, White privilege, etc.)

- In meetings or gatherings my ideas or comments are recognized.
- I can go out to a place of business, a restaurant, or an event and not worry about accessibility.
- I can go to a restaurant or a movie and not need someone to read the menu or list of showings.
- I can travel, purchase items, go out for entertainment (i.e., have financial resources) without concern about how I will purchase the necessities for daily living.
- I can hold my partner's hand in social contexts without concern.
- I can attend the church or place of worship I desire.
- I can speak for myself as an individual and not feel like I am representing a group of people with my same skin color (or gender, religion, etc.).

Discrimination

The second concept we want to introduce is discrimination, which refers to a behavior that usually stems from prejudiced feelings or thoughts and results in denying "individuals or groups of people equality of treatment" (Blumenfeld & Raymond, 2000, p. 22). In our opening story, Cella and Val – as Black people – were both were targets of discrimination (not being acknowledged or seen – treated as if they were invisible) while White people just behind them were recipients of respect (acknowledged and seen). When discrimination takes place on a larger scale, we talk about oppression, which refers to "the systematic, institutionalized mistreatment of one group of people by another" (Lustig & Koester, 1999, p. 159).

The following example is something that happened in Sharon's family the very week we were writing this chapter, and addresses another type of privilege (male privilege) and discrimination:

> Bobby (9 years old) said to me (Sharon), "Mom, when we (he and his sister Taya, 8 years old) go over to the neighbor's house to see if Kenny can play, Gene always says, 'Bobby's at the door.' He doesn't say anything about Taya." I asked Bobby why he thought Gene didn't mention Taya when he announced who was at the door. Bobby said he thought it was that Gene didn't like Taya.

I responded, "That might be true. It might also be that he doesn't see Taya as 'counting' or deserving notice." The assumption might be that Taya is "invisible" to Gene because of her gender. Whether or not that is Gene's intent, one covert message to Taya may be, "Bobby, you're visible and important to recognize (male privilege) and Taya, you're invisible and don't count."

In all three incidents, the harm was overt and personal. All three individuals were made aware of their "invisibility" by another individual. There was also some indirect or covert harm that Sharon participated in as she interacted with Cella. Although Sharon's words to Cella were ones of acknowledgement and understanding, her underlying thoughts were of disbelief. She saw Cella as being overly sensitive to what she thought was an obvious misunderstanding on Cella's part. Sharon was inadvertently and ignorantly colluding with the person behind the counter who saw Cella as invisible. Sharon couldn't see the issue because she had been "conditioned into oblivion about its existence" (McIntosh, 1990, p. 31).

When we overcome our conditioned oblivion to our own points of privilege, we may be more able to offer the best therapy to our clients. We will be able more fully to really hear, empathize with, and respect some of our clients' experiences of discrimination and oppression and thereby acknowledge, rather than discount, their experience (Furman, 2005; Tuason, 2005).

Harm can also be societal, and it can happen in neighborhoods, large systems, organizations, and institutions. In the world of psychotherapy, groups of people have been overlooked, devalued, and disrespected because of being different from the "norm" or from the dominant culture.

Journal Entry: *Don't Judge a Book by Its Cover*

Think of a time when you or another person close to you was ignored, devalued, or prejudged because of age, gender, disability, beliefs (spiritual or political), language or speech, or choice of partner (same gender, skin color difference, another issue of difference). Who was doing the ignoring, devaluing, prejudging? How did it feel? What were the resulting behaviors?

Social Responsibility

We have moral and ethical obligations to treat individual people (co-workers, employees, friends, etc.) fairly and ethically. We fulfill our obligations by our actions toward these individuals. We can call this *individual responsibility*. Social responsibility has more to do with our ethical obligations to help *society* treat individuals in moral ways.

Recognizing our points of privilege and the potential for discrimination naturally lead us to considerations of social responsibility. In talking about privilege, McIntosh (1990) states it this way: "Describing … privilege makes one newly accountable. As we in women's studies work to reveal male privilege and ask men to give up some of their power, so one who writes about having White privilege must ask, 'Having described it, what will I do to lessen or end it?' " (p. 31). Working toward helping society behave ethically towards its members, rather than only behaving ethically ourselves, is what we mean by social responsibility. Social responsibility is a "duty owed to society at large" (Clark, 1993, p. 307) and includes a duty to question and oppose community standards that work against promoting human welfare.

One way to fulfill our social responsibility is to work for *social justice*, which refers to fair treatment, or fair opportunity, for all individuals in society. Working for social justice might mean lobbying legislatures for laws that ensure equal access to such societal benefits as housing and health care. One of those societal benefits might be psychotherapy. Kitchener (2000) writes:

> The question of whether psychological services [including psychotherapy] are luxuries to be enjoyed by the wealthy or necessities that all people should be able to use is one of social justice … the respect due to all people, regardless of their ethnicity, gender, social class or whether they are differently abled, are owed fair treatment … Acting in a socially responsible way would include an ethical duty to challenge injustice when it exists. (pp. 185–186)

As professionals in the field of psychotherapy, we would likely agree that psychotherapy should be available to all and that when we see an injustice, the ethical thing to do is stand up and make some noise.

Psychotherapy, because it so clearly involves face-to-face interactions, may be seen as a way to fulfill our individual responsibilities. But many psychotherapists want to "change the world" by being a therapist. How might our individual and social responsibilities fit together? We invite you to think about your own sense of social responsibility in the context of your study of psychotherapy.

Journal Entry: *Social Responsibility and Motivations*

What is your social responsibility and how does this issue relate to your motivations for being a psychotherapist? Take a moment to look back at the exercise in chapter 1 where you identified or listed your motivations for being a psychotherapist. As you review this list, which motivations suggest a call to promoting or improving the welfare of humans? Which ones represent a mixed picture – addressing the call to help individuals as well as the call to social responsibility? Which ones are more exclusively individual in nature? How might you fulfill both your individual and social responsibility by being a psychotherapist?

In this chapter, we've looked at several issues that are part of your ethical culture of origin. For some of you, this may have been an uncomfortable chapter to read. Looking at our points of privilege is hard work. Let us emphasize a couple of things about this journey we are all on. First, coming to know our points of privilege is a process and increasing our awareness in this area is the first step. Second, you are not alone in this journey. We are all on the same journey, although we might have different points of privilege, experience different types of discrimination and oppression, and be at different points along the way. Third, as we become more aware, our efforts to be more socially responsible can be actualized more effectively. Finally, don't expect to be perfect in this journey. Be willing to have the difficult dialogues, hear the feedback from others along the way, own what is yours but don't punish yourself for mistakes and missteps along the way. Remember, this work is a process. Understanding privilege, oppression, and social responsibility, along with your values, virtues, and motivations, gives you a firm foundation on which to build your professionals identity. We are ready now to explore the ethical acculturation process and the culture of psychotherapy.

3

The Process of Acculturation
Developing Your Professional Ethical Identity

Now that you have a sense of the basic moral equipment you are working with, we discuss in more detail the process of moving into the culture of psychotherapy. How do we do that? Let's start with an activity with several scenes and variations. For this activity, we suggest you read all the parts and then respond to aspects of the scenarios and variations that strike you.

Food for Thought: *On the Street Where You Live*

Scenario 1   Imagine that it is a beautiful day. You've launched your new career as a psychotherapist and your case load is growing. Life is good. As you walk down a street not far from where you live, a small group of people come around the corner. You instantly recognize one of the folks; it is Brandon, one of your best friends. Your hand shoots up for a big wave, you smile and call out a friendly "Hello."

Scenario 2   Imagine that it is a beautiful day. You've launched your new career as a psychotherapist and your case load is growing. Life is good. As you walk down a street not far from where you live, a small group of people come around the corner. You instantly recognize one of the folks as Charlie. In that same split second you start to smile and lift your hand to wave "Hello" but stop it midair. You stop because Charlie is a client of yours. You stop to think.

In Scenario 1, what went through your mind as you recognized Brandon? What did you think about before you said hello? Was there even the thought not to wave and say hello? What would it have felt like if you had walked by Brandon without saying anything?

In Scenario 2, what went through your mind as you recognized Charlie? What caused you to stop your wave? What are your choices as the two of you walk toward each other on the street?

Variation on Scenario 2   Eliza, an acquaintance of yours and another person in the small group, sees you say hello to Charlie. Later that day at a neighborhood meeting Eliza comes up to you and says, "Charlie is one of my best friends. I didn't know the two of you know each other. How do *you* know Charlie?" How do you respond?

Variation on Scenario 1   You and Brandon are walking down the street and somebody gives Brandon a big hello. You ask, "Who was that?" In fact, that person is Brandon's therapist but you don't know that. What might happen?

Scenario 3   It is another beautiful day. Your career as a psychotherapist is going well. Your personal life, however, is a different story. You've recently begun working with a psychotherapist. As you're walking down the street, your therapist appears from around the corner. He gives you a big "Hello!" as he walks by. How do you feel? How do you respond?

Variation on Scenario 3   As he walks away, you hear his walking companion ask him, "Who was that?" How do you feel? How do you hope he responds to the question?

Variation on Scenario 3   You are walking with a business associate who asks you, "Who was that?" How do you feel? How do you respond?

We hope that in Scenario 1 you had no problem deciding to say hello to your friend. Caring people do that with friends, acquaintances, and sometimes even strangers. However, as a psychotherapist you have to think more carefully about even these natural social interactions and here's why: Clients may feel awkward at being greeted by their therapist, and such a greeting may violate *contact confidentiality* (Ahia & Martin, 1993; see chapter 6). That is, it may communicate to others the private fact that a person is a client.

When we enter the culture of psychotherapy, some of these typical human interactions that express our basic values and motivations don't work the same as in the everyday social interactions we have with our friends. It can be a strange and uncomfortable experience to see some-body on the street with whom we've worked, *intimately* in a therapeutic way, and not acknowledge their existence, even by a wink. This internal discomfort may cause what we will discuss later as *acculturation stress*.

Here's another variation on this story, told by Sharon:

> We have a counseling lab at Colorado State University for our master's-level students. Our students are videotaped working with volunteer clients, most of whom are college students. A couple of years ago I'm supervising a student and she's working with this client and they are doing good work. A couple of months later, after the semester is over, I see this former client on campus. Immediately I recognize him, but I didn't stop to think how I recognize him. I just know that I recognize him. With my friendly side in full gear I say, "Hi." Not just a nondescript "Hi" like I don't know you, but more like, "Hi! How's it goin'?" Then I remember how I know him and realize that he has no clue as to why I am so friendly! In this case, he could be wondering whether I am just an overly friendly person, whether I am slightly strange, or even whether I am coming onto him. He had no way of knowing that I had a professional rela-tionship with him as my student's supervisor!

Let's assume that this former client was with a friend and the friend asked, "Who was that?" In this case the former client could genuinely say, "I don't know. Maybe I look like someone else she knows. I've never seen her before." This would be true; he hadn't seen Sharon before. As a supervisor, Sharon had seen a lot of him and knew a whole lot about his life from watching taped counseling sessions. On the other hand, if Sharon had been this person's therapist and given him that big hello, it could have caused him some unnecessary discomfort and embarrassment. He would have three options of how to respond to his friend: choose to tell a lie, choose to tell the truth, or choose to ignore his friend's question. None of these options may feel real good.

In the social environment, being a therapist probably means being more conscious of social interactions. It might mean pausing, even if just for a second, and asking, "How do I know this person?" We might have to hesitate when we say hello. This is one of the costs of being a professional. We have to take extra steps to be careful in social situations in which people in other professions can interact without a second thought. We need to adapt our pre-existing moral sense to the expectations of our new profession.

Of course, many of these types of decisions get easier and more routine as we go along. But let's look at another and possibly more conflicted example.

Journal Entry: *Friends and/or Colleagues*

You and your friend both get a job in which you are counseling high school students in an after-school program. The program has a strict policy against drinking or drug use among both students and staff members, and your friend – who is now also your colleague – is showing up for work high or hung over.

- How do you feel about your friend's decision to violate the school's policy?
- Do you think you need to report your friend?
  - If yes, why?
  - If no, why not?
- What if you knew that your friend was definitely harming students by coming to work in this condition?
- Would your answer be different from before?
  - If yes, why?
  - If no, why not?
- What values drive your decisions?
- How do you feel about your decisions?
- What if you knew it was mandatory to report this type of behavior by a fellow colleague – would that change your answer?

- If you decided you needed to report your friend, how did you imagine yourself actually taking the necessary steps to action?

Variation: What if the colleague wasn't your friend?

- How do you feel about your colleague's decision?
- Do you decide to report your colleague for violating agency policy?
  - If yes, why?
  - If not, why not?
- What if you knew this person was definitely harming students by coming to work in these conditions?
- What values drive your decisions?
- How do you feel about your decisions?
- If you decided you needed to report your colleague, how did you imagine yourself actually taking the necessary steps to action?

There are research data to suggest that many graduate students and practicing psychologists would not behave ethically even when they know they should (Bernard & Jara, 1986; Bernard, Murphy, & Little, 1987). It appears as though personal values such as friendship and loyalty get in the way of our professional obligations (Betan & Stanton, 1999), perhaps by making us less objective in our judgments or by weakening our moral courage to uphold our professional responsibility. Whether or not you chose to report your friend's behavior, you might be feeling conflicted, guilty, and/or disloyal. Once again, we need to adapt our pre-existing moral sense to the expectations of our new profession. Let's look more deeply into this process, which we call *ethical acculturation*.

The Process of Ethical Acculturation

John Berry is a cross-cultural psychologist at Queen's University. He and his colleagues (Berry, 1980, 2003; Berry & Kim, 1988; Berry & Sam, 1997) have written extensively about psychological acculturation, the process that immigrants, refugees, sojourners, and others go through when they adapt to a new culture. In this sense, acculturation is defined as "a set of internal psychological outcomes including a clear sense of personal and cultural identity, good mental health, and the achievement of personal satisfaction in the new cultural context" (Berry & Sam, 1997, p. 299). Handelsman, Gottlieb, and Knapp (2005) adapted Berry's definition to the notion of ethical acculturation by substituting the word "ethical" for the word "cultural" in this definition.

As we have seen, when we acculturate to the psychotherapy profession we cannot express many of our moral virtues (e.g., compassion) in the same ways as before. Also, we may have to develop new virtues such as those surrounding informed consent (e.g., therapeutically informative). As Grater (1985) suggested, "To a significant extent the trainee learns to replace social patterns of interacting with therapeutic responses" (p. 606). But the process of acculturation is more complicated than merely replacing one set of values, behaviors, or virtues with another. Our pre-existing moral senses are not meant to be replaced in a wholesale fashion; rather, the best outcome is when our ethics of origin are refined, adapted, and integrated with those of the culture of psychotherapy.

Berry (Berry & Sam, 1997) discussed two major dimensions of acculturation: (a) maintenance and (b) contact and participation. Applied to ethical acculturation, maintenance refers to how much of our personal moral sense we bring with us, as it were, to the new culture. As Berry and Sam (1997) state, the task of maintenance is addressed by the person exploring the following question: "Is it considered to be of value to maintain cultural [ethical, moral] identity and characteristics?" (p. 296). As you review your motivations, values, and virtues – and their expressions – you will notice that some of them you cannot live without, some you can implement in different ways, and some (like saying "hello" to everybody you know) can be discarded.

Contact and participation, the second dimension, refers to how much we identify with and adopt the traditions, values, and behaviors of our new culture. As you deepen your study of psychotherapy, you will discover more and more aspects of the culture that are different from your expectations and different from how you have engaged in relationships before. In the next activity we give you an opportunity to explore some initial impressions and experiences of entering the psychotherapy culture.

Journal Entry: *Surprise, Surprise*

We've adapted the following questions from Handelsman et al., 2005 (p. 62): In studying your discipline, what is the most counterintuitive, shocking, or surprising professional activity that you have learned about so far? What didn't you expect about being or becoming a psychotherapist? What feelings have you experienced, positively and negatively, about the culture of psychotherapy? You can answer these with general comments, or by telling stories about those times when you felt either that you had signed up for something you didn't bargain for, you felt like you made a mistake, or you simply felt like a stranger in a strange land.

Your reflections in this journal entry constitute your knowledge, thus far, of the ethical culture of psychotherapy. Later in this book, we shall explore the major ethical elements of this culture, such as boundaries, confidentiality, and informed consent.

Four Strategies of Acculturation

If we think of the two dimensions – (a) maintenance and (b) contact and participation – as variables along which one can be relatively high or low, we see the possibility of four alternatives for acculturation choices. We can be high on both maintenance and contact, low on both dimensions, or high on one and low on the other (see Figure 3.1). "*Attitudes* towards these four alternatives, and actual *behaviors* exhibiting them, together constitute an individual's acculturation *strategy*" (Berry & Sam, 1997, p. 297, emphases in original). We're ready to take a look at each of the four types of strategies applied to ethical acculturation.

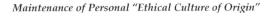

Maintenance of Personal "Ethical Culture of Origin"

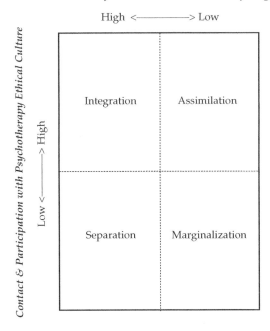

Figure 3.1 Strategies of ethical acculturation (adapted from Handelsman, Gottlieb, & Knapp, 2005)

Integration

If we choose both to maintain our personal moral sense and adopt elements of the culture of psychotherapy, we are choosing the strategy of integration. Integration can occur in different ways: upholding a personal value that overlaps with a professional value; modifying the expression of a personal value; creating and internalizing a new value; and/or reorganizing or reprioritizing our values. The following paragraphs illustrate each of these options.

Sometimes the integration strategy involves a relatively simple overlapping of our personal moral sense and values with the values of the professional culture. For example, we may hold this value: "When people we care about are in distress, we give them our undivided attention." This value works for our close friends, professional colleagues, and psychotherapy clients.

However, because psychotherapy is a unique kind of relationship, a simple overlap of values and their expression is less frequent than we might think. Integration more often means that we need to modify the expression of existing values. For example, remember the previous scenario where we're walking down the street and notice our client coming toward us? We might understand that showing respect to friends means saying hello, but showing respect to clients means honoring their privacy. When we honor their right to privacy we can feel good about our interaction with our client even though we did not say hello. We have thus upheld the personal value of respect and the professional value of confidentiality (among others).

Another example of modifying the expression of values concerns privacy, which we discuss in great detail in chapter 6. With our friends, we respect their privacy by not talking about them to strangers, but it may be perfectly acceptable to talk about our friends to our spouses, partners, or closest friends. However, when the personal value of privacy is integrated with the professional value of confidentiality, we refrain from talking about our clients to *anybody*, even our partners, closest friends, and relatives.

A third example of modifying our expression of values might be how and when we give advice. Giving advice to friends might be an expression of our concern and compassion. In psychotherapy, however, one very common goal is to have clients become more able and willing to deliberate and make decisions for themselves. In the psychotherapy relationship, demonstrating concern and compassion would mean *not* giving advice. (We will revisit issues around advice giving in chapter 5.)

As we can see, sometimes integration means adapting our behavior to express pre-existing values in a new context. However, there will be other times when we need to create and internalize entirely new values. For some of us, privacy is not really an issue among friends. We might have a circle of friends and it is perfectly acceptable to talk within that circle about any of the conversations we have with any of our friends. In the psychotherapy culture, we need an entirely new concept of confidentiality: In the psychotherapy relationship, the information that is shared with you and by you is *not* yours to disclose outside of the relationship. The ownership of clients' information remains with clients, who must give permission, barring any exceptions to confidentiality addressed in chapter 6, for you to share it with anybody else.

Another new concept in the psychotherapy profession that we need to adapt to has to do with being honest or sharing information about what we do and who we are. In psychotherapy this is called *informed consent* (see chapter 7). In friendship we typically do not ask explicit permission of people to become their friend but discover how important it is to be honest and open as the relationship grows. But in psychotherapy the process is different. There is a kind of laying all the cards out on the table – via the informed consent process – where we share information about ourselves as a professional and ask clients explicitly if they wish to become our clients.

Another variation of the integration strategy is to reorganize our values – we elevate the relative importance of some of our values or create a higher value that helps us adapt to our psychotherapeutic roles. For example, you might consider loyalty and compassion to be your highest values – after all, they are key elements of a good friendship. Loyalty and compassion in friendship involve such behaviors as self-disclosure, saying hello when you meet your friend on the street, lending or receiving money when either of you are in need, or being your friend's first insurance client.

As a professional psychotherapist, however, your implementation of your values such as loyalty and compassion will revolve around confidentiality, consent, and maintaining clear boundaries. Demonstrating these values typically involves behaviors like little to no self-disclosing to clients, *not* initiating a social interaction with a client in a public setting, *not* entering into business arrangements with clients, and *not* doing therapy with those with whom you have another relationship. With all these constraints, we might conclude that to be a therapist means not showing or experiencing compassion. If this thought has crossed your mind, you might be thinking, "What am I doing in this profession? I am all about people and being compassionate."

The solution to this dilemma – or acculturation crisis (Berry & Kim, 1988; see p. 61) – is realizing that the integration strategy doesn't negate the value of compassion; rather, it encourages us to put the value of *respect* at the top of our values hierarchy in our professional life. Knowing we are upholding the value of respect allows us to retain a sense of consistency across situations. Thus, integration strategies help us recognize and possibly reduce at least to some extent the tension between our personal and professional roles and identities. Integration means that we can read the ethical standards of our profession and think, "I understand the values behind the rules and I can heartily endorse those values. I'll find ethical ways to reduce the inevitable tension between my personal values and those of my new profession." It is possible that an integration strategy allows us to more easily employ the four components of Rest's model of moral behavior (Gilley, Anderson, & Gilley, 2008).

In terms of psychological acculturation, Berry and his colleagues conclude, "Evidence strongly supports a positive correlation between the use of this strategy and good psychological adaptation during acculturation" (Berry & Sam, 1997, p. 298). We believe that making the effort to integrate our personal and professional ethics will lead to good *ethical* adaptation, which gives us the best chance of becoming and staying ethically excellent psychotherapists.

Before we leave this section on integration, we need to make two points very clear: First, integration does not mean bending the rules to fit our personalities. Rather, integration has more to do with how we approach these rules. Anderson, Wagoner, and Moore (2006) state it this way:

> The more the individual can adapt to the new culture ... with its values, philosophy, and traditions – while retraining aspects of one's ethics of origin or personal ethics, the better the fit, and the more likely the individual is to have a coherent professional ethical identity. (p. 48)

Second, even when we use integration strategies and we behave in ethically excellent ways, we may not always feel good! The joy and fulfillment of behaving ethically is sometimes overshadowed by unpleasantness engendered by what philosophers call the wrong-making features of many actions – those aspects that are not ethically perfect because of values conflicts or other considerations. For example, when we report colleagues for unprofessional behavior we feel bad that their careers and relationships may suffer. We may also feel conflicted when we've behaved consistently with our professional role even as we are aware of our limitations: not being able to help as much as we'd like, not being able to fully pursue our interests, etc. For example, we might be convinced that entering into a business partnership with a client would be beneficial to everyone involved, but we know that this would be an unethical multiple relationship (see chapter 5).

Assimilation

We might believe that being a psychotherapist is *so* different from any other role we play that we might as well build our professional self from scratch. Thus, we might actively jettison, or simply lose track of, our own moral sense and we totally adopt the ethical values and traditions of psychotherapy as our sole source of professional guidance. This is an extreme of the strategy of *assimilation*.

You might be thinking, "What's wrong with assimilation? Aren't I supposed to follow the rules of the profession?" To those of you thinking this, we applaud your motivation and your dedication to the profession. Indeed, to the observer, many assimilation behaviors would look identical to integration behaviors. However, just following the rules to the letter is not enough to be a professional. In addition, having a degree, professional license, nicely furnished office, business attire, does not automatically equal professionalism. "These outward signs are meaningless and potentially harmful without a firm personal grounding in and appreciation for the ethics and value traditions of the professional culture" (Handelsman et al., 2005, p. 61).

In the short term, assimilation strategies might be better than others as we strive toward integration. For example, it is a pretty good idea for new psychotherapists to maintain client confidentiality even if they don't yet feel the connection between that behavior and their own moral sense. However, if you maintain this strategy over time you might become alienated from the profession because you are following rules without an optimal level of personal involvement. The rules become hollow because you feel little or no personal investment in either the rules or their underlying values. As ethical decisions become more difficult (remember the journal entry with your hypothetical friend/colleague using drugs), you may find it harder to make the subtle judgments that are required. In a sense, you will only have half of the ethical tools you need to achieve ethical excellence. Another risk is that your new professional sensibilities spill over into your non-therapy relationships. You may find, for example, that you feel the need to recommend or provide professional help to every person you meet at social gatherings.

Consider this scenario: You come home from a day of therapy and your spouse asks, "How'd it go today?" You know that you are supposed to keep client information confidential and you are determined to obey that rule so you reply, "I'm sorry, I'm not allowed to say." Your spouse responds, "But I'm your spouse; you're supposed to share about your day with me!" And they have a point! If you choose an extreme assimilation strategy, you might hold your ground and refuse to discuss your work. But this response is based on a skewed, half-informed understanding of the rules and their applications.

In contrast, an integration strategy might lead you to keep in mind the rules about confidentiality but also appreciate your values about close human relationships. Thus, you might choose to share some of your feelings without violating client confidentiality: "Well the day started well; my first couple of sessions felt really good and this was rewarding – like I really got a chance to do what I was trained to do. But in the afternoon I felt like I struggled more in my sessions. As a result, I was pretty frustrated by the end of the day." Notice that your partner will not know who your clients are or the clients' part of the therapy, but can stay in touch with who *you* are and how the day was.

We hope this scenario illustrates our point that integration does not mean bending the rules; rather, true integration into the professional culture has to do with how we handle the rules. Observers may not be able to tell if we're using assimilation or integration strategies, because from the outside they might look like identical adherence to the rules. The differences will be internal: therapists choosing integration strategies have found areas of overlap between what they value personally and what they must do professionally. They feel more comfortable with the tensions that may exist between these two spheres.

Separation

If we choose to maintain our personal moral sense but do not identify with the culture of psychotherapy, we are choosing the strategy of separation. Many beginning students of psychotherapy choose separation strategies in their ethical deliberations because they do not yet know about the culture of therapy (see chapter 4). They are relying on their personal frameworks for how relationships work and/or see the rules as limiting or confining. They have not yet begun to see the ethical rules as being grounded in ethical principles which provide a firm foundation for ethical choices.

Again, imagine being at the dinner table with your partner, who asks you how it went today. You feel that unburdening yourself after a difficult day would be a mentally healthy thing to do. It would make you feel better. It would even help you get back into the office tomorrow and have a better day. Indeed, you'd be a better therapist! So you start,

> "Well, David and Eleanor's sessions went quite well. You remember Eleanor – she's the accountant who was getting anxious about her upcoming exams? Thank goodness, she's doing much better. But in the afternoon, Alan's session was tough. He works downtown, you know, where our insurance woman's office is – the next office. Anyway, his daughter Sarah isn't doing well at school. Sarah just started Rutland Elementary School, where our Jason's going to go next year …"

You feel so much better after sharing about your whole day. And you are sure your clients wouldn't mind you talking about them to your partner because, after all, it's really for their own benefit.

In this situation you are using a separation strategy. You are acting on your preexisting moral sense (Kitchener, 2000), including doing good for clients based only on your own moral guides and handling your partnership well because you value sharing in the relationship, and see this as a way of taking care of yourself. In making these decisions, however, you are not valuing the demands of the professional principle of confidentiality and the client's right to privacy. These behaviors violate the privacy of your client and are unethical.

Separation may show itself when the personal values of clients conflict with your own personal values and needs. For example, family members, friends, financial planners, religious advisors, and others may not have any prohibitions against condemning their friends' or clients' plans to get a divorce, have an affair, marry a person with another skin color, vote Libertarian, marry their childhood sweetheart, not have children, buy an extended warranty on their car, or listen to jazz. But as a therapist you are expected to not impose your personal values on your clients. Your task is to encourage clients to live the life they need to live themselves, not the life you want for them.

One lens with which we view the world is the lens of individuality. With friendships and other relationships, we come to value the uniqueness of each individual – we might treat each of our friends differently because of who they are to us. Clinically, we are also taught by most schools of therapy to keep in mind the uniqueness of each client. However, when we come to ethics we need to appreciate that some values and behaviors are relatively absolute. For example, each client we see is worthy of equal respect because they are equally human. Boundaries need to be respected no matter what the characteristics of individual clients.

Bucher and Stelling (1977) conducted a longitudinal study of professional training programs in internal medicine, psychiatry, and biochemistry. In the report of their study they discussed what they called *socialization failures*, which are students who did not fit the mold of the training program. Among the characteristics of these socialization failures was a rigid commitment to a pre-existing value orientation. We might guess that these students adopted separation strategies and, although they had good intentions for their future profession, they never identified with their new professional cultures. It is important to realize that good intentions are not enough to assure good professional practice. As Handelsman et al. (2005) said:

> Although they may have a very strong personal code of ethics and be very well intentioned, these students may also be unaware of the potential harm that may come from acting on a set of principles or virtues that are inconsistent with the professional context (p. 61).

In light of all this discussion, it might appear that ethical rules may take away some of the choices we thought we had. When you come across ethical standards that don't strike you as right or beneficial to the client, you may think of them as stupid little rules and therefore not necessary to follow. Edging toward integration, however, means that we appreciate the consistency that ethical rules and guidelines provide which helps us treat clients ethically. This consistency actually provides the necessary conditions under which we can learn about and empathize with the uniqueness of our clients. If your first reaction is to minimize the importance of the ethical guidelines, we would encourage you to think of these standards in these ways:

- Perhaps they are professional implementations of higher values that you actually have in common with the culture of psychotherapy.
- They are an opportunity for you to see if you can articulate your own values, virtues, and motivations along with the values,

traditions, and principles that underlie the standard. Then, you are on your way to integrating your values, traditions, and principles with the culture of psychotherapy.

- They are, ironically perhaps, the key to your future fulfillment as an ethically excellent psychotherapist! If followed from true understanding and appreciation, they will produce ethical excellence. They are an opportunity to explore a positive ethical approach: You can take the opportunity to see how you can achieve higher purposes by going beyond what the rule says is the minimum. Here's an example: Some states require informing clients that sex between clients and therapists is a crime. At the very least, you could reproduce the statute in your informed consent statement (see chapter 7) and ask the client to read it and sign a document that they have read the relevant statute. Or you could use this "disclosure rule" as a stimulus to talk with clients about a range of topics, including a variety of the boundaries of the therapy relationship (see chapter 5).

Marginalization

"Those exhibiting marginalization will obey ethical standards out of personal convenience rather than a sense of moral commitment" (Handelsman et al., 2005, p. 61). Marginalization is basically the worst of both worlds. We do not identify with our new culture and we also lose sight of our own moral sense. Marginalization is similar to a rudderless ship on the sea – drifting along with no mechanism to guide its course (Gilley, Anderson, & Gilley, 2008).

Marginalization can be a temporary strategy. We may begin our training thinking that we can simply adopt a professional persona, but we are still unaware of what the new culture entails. As a result, we make mistakes, like suggesting specific courses of action for our clients simply because they're expedient or would somehow benefit us.

Sometimes we may get dislodged from our moral compasses when we are impaired in some way. Going through a divorce or other relationship crisis, losing support groups when we move, or abusing drugs or alcohol are all examples of times when we might choose marginalization. We might falsify work records to secure more money, or we might "judge" that it's best for a couple we are seeing to split up, secretly hoping that this could lead to a social or romantic relationship with one member of the couple. These are behaviors that are clearly wrong professionally, and we hope you would judge them as wrong according to your own intuitive moral sense.

Journal Entry: *Acculturation Strategies*

We just spent some time describing each of the acculturation strategies. As you were reading you might have thought, "Wow, I remember when I ..." or "You know, now I understand why ..." In this entry, write down some of those thoughts. Try and think of times when your behavior or attitude (or the behavior or attitude of someone you observed) demonstrates each one of the four strategies.

We imagine that you will be (or have been) a psychotherapist who strives to choose integration strategies and succeeds most of the time. However, there will be times when you will not choose integration. When that's the case, which strategy are you most likely to choose? Are you most likely to slip into assimilation strategies (e.g., "Let me just follow the rules to protect myself even though I really don't see the value."); separation strategies (e.g., "I'm a nice person, so what I do will naturally be therapeutic"); or marginalization strategies (e.g., "What's the use of even trying to do the right thing?!")?

Acculturation Stress

Acculturation stress refers to the difficulties we may face as we adapt to being a psychotherapist. As we've touched on earlier, acculturation stress can arise when we need to stop and think before we act because our response as a professional needs to be different than that as a friend.

Acculturation stress can start early in our careers. For example, one source of stress is that the culture of psychotherapy and your training are imperfect. You may find, for example, that your professors, supervisors, and others you thought would be perfect role models may not be so perfect (Glaser & Thorpe, 1986; Hammel, Olkin, & Taube, 1996; Branstetter & Handelsman, 2000).

Another example of acculturation stress: Not every professional you meet will be comfortable talking about ethical issues. Here are just two cases. Some psychotherapists find it difficult to admit to others that they have had sexual feelings for clients (see Pope, Sonne, & Greene, 2006). Other psychotherapists may be quick to interpret a question about their ethics as an accusation of misbehavior and they may experience your inquiry about the ethical rationale for their behavior as an ethical insult (Veatch & Sollitto, 1976).

In addition, you may also find that psychotherapy does not help all who seek services or not to the extent you would like. It may be a new realization for you that problems for which people seek psychotherapy are not easily solved! Some clients, for example, will have thought of virtually all of the solutions that occur to you and already have many reasons why such solutions won't work.

Food for Thought: *Acculturation Stress*

Imagine the following scenario: The clinical director of the mental health center calls and offers you a job. She mentions that the clincher for her in you getting the job was your comment about wanting to help people since you were very young. You are confident that you will do well, but even so you are a little nervous. The night before your first day on the job you dream about the most unpleasant type of person you've ever known or heard about. This person triggers feelings of anger and disgust any time you think about them. The next day, your very first client is a person who in some important way reminds you of the person in your dream. They look like the person, they're a member of the same group as the person, and they have the same attitudes. What do you think? How do you feel? What are your options? What would you do if you had no constraints? What do you do?

Now put yourself in the role of the client, and the therapist has these feelings toward you. What are you expecting from this therapist? How would you react if they did what you were considering as the therapist?

Acculturation stress can also involve a mismatch between your strengths and the skills required of a psychotherapist. These are inevitable because no one person can ever master all the skills involved in all types of psychotherapy with all types of clients. For example, you may be a problem-solver by nature and feel impatient with friends and colleagues who like to mull over options, reflect, and deliberate before taking action. Your problem-solving approach may work very well in your social relationships, in your other jobs (as a stockbroker, ski instructor, software developer), and with your recreational activities. In psychotherapy, quick problem-solving is the exception rather than the rule and you may find yourself challenged to expand your repertoire of helping behaviors and attitudes.

The gulf between the skills, virtues, values, and motivations you bring and those required of psychotherapists is similar to what Berry and Sam (1997) called *cultural distance* (p. 307). If the distance between the two cultures, in this case your ethical traditions and those of psychotherapy, is very great, you may need to engage in some *cultural shedding*, which Berry and Sam defined as "the *un*learning of aspects of one's previous repertoire that are no longer appropriate" (p. 298).

If you are coming into the psychotherapy profession after having been in another profession, such as law, medicine, or even other mental health activities, your cultural shedding may be especially stressful. You may find that skills you thought would be helpful are not. Handelsman et al. (2005) present the following example:

> One trainee had previously worked as a counselor in a domestic abuse shelter, where it was common for counselors to engage in substantial self-disclosure, especially about their own abuse backgrounds. She initially resented the admonition that her self-disclosures as a psychologist had to be more selective and carefully timed. (p. 63)

Coming from other professions may also be stressful because of the loss of status, power, or prestige. As Berry and Kim (1988) state: "One's 'entry status' into the larger society [psychotherapy] is often lower than one's 'departure status' from the home society" (p. 216).

Trying to understand the ethical standards which are often vague and contradictory can prompt acculturation stress. When our students have asked for an answer to an ethical issue, on more than one occasion we've responded with, "It depends." Such ambiguities or seeming contradictions happen to be one of the most frustrating features of the profession for many of our students. For example, psychotherapists are required to maintain confidentiality but also to report child abuse. In addition, psychotherapists are required to report their clients' threats of physical harm against others, but not report the fact that a client has committed a crime in the past (see chapter 6). At these times, the stress we face may feel really awful. "If conflict and tension do appear, a highly stressful *crisis* phase may then occur, in which the conflict comes to a head, and a resolution is required" (Berry & Kim, 1988, p. 210).

Acculturation Stress in Professional and Personal Relationships

Acculturation is an all-encompassing phenomenon, not just a professional one. Before we continue this discussion, we'd like you to read and respond to the following food for thought.

Food for Thought: *More Acculturation Stress*

Think about some of the circumstances in your life that have changed along with entering a psychotherapy training program. These circumstances can be economic changes; less family and other support; attitude changes toward you among your friends and relations; or adjustments you've had to make to a new set of friends, professors, colleagues, etc. What would make some of these stresses easier? What types of circumstances would be too stressful for you?

The acculturation process changes both our professional relationships and our personal ones. By adopting new values and reorienting the ones we have, we inevitably make and experience shifts in our personal relationships. These shifts also occur because people treat us differently. The uncomfortable news is that people close to us may struggle with the change. On the other hand, changes in both types of relationships can be quite positive. With the broader perspective that comes from integration, we may find that we can develop a range of skills that are helpful in all our relationships.

How to Deal with Acculturation Stress

Remember the treadmill analogy in chapter 1? Remember how we encouraged you to relax and not make any premature decisions about your fit with the profession or get overwhelmed with all the cultural changes that lay in front of you? Again, we want you to relax and consider the following guides – "troubleshooting" steps – as you explore who you are in this professional culture:

- Keep learning. Remember that learning to become ethically excellent is not an event that happens in 10 or 16 weeks; it is a lifelong process (Handelsman, 2001b). Ethical acculturation never stops! You start now, but over the course of your professional life you will change and the professional culture will change. For example, it wasn't that long ago when managed care didn't exist, Prozac didn't exist, and even family therapy didn't exist. We encourage you to be open to exploration of yourself and the profession.
- Keep your eyes open. You may start with simple notions, but don't stop there. For example, "Put your clients' needs above your own" is a nice platitude to keep in mind, but reality happens. Something's got to give when your client calls in crisis and needs to see you and at the same time you are sitting in the emergency room receiving area with your sick child. Remember that psychotherapy, ethics, clients and their problems, and you and your life are more complex than it might first appear.
- Keep your mind open. If you are not "getting it" when your professors, supervisors, or colleagues talk with you about ethical

requirements, do not immediately assume that you are an unethical person or cannot become an ethical therapist. At the same time, don't assume that your professors and supervisors are totally off the wall. We encourage you to take some time to think through the acculturation stress you are facing and explore a variety of avenues that will help you choose integration strategies. Find some very good ethical role models and see what they have to offer. Be especially cognizant of their advice when you feel most stressed. But keep your mind open and remember that nobody's perfect.

- Keep your mouth open! By this we mean that you should develop an ethical support network of professors, colleagues, fellow students, and even folks in other professions. The more you can get into the habit of seeing the professional world in terms of ethics, the smoother your acculturation will be.
- Keep your heart open. Give yourself some time to develop a full range of ethical reasoning and reflecting skills. Strive for perfection, but don't be too hard on yourself when it doesn't quite happen. Keep a sense of perspective and endeavor to become more fully human as you become more fully professional.

Mismatch with the Profession?

As we were writing this first part of the book, we talked a lot about having a section that raises the possibility that psychotherapy may not be the profession for you. We questioned ourselves about where and how to address the issue. We decided to be honest and not pull any punches. After all, taking a positive approach doesn't mean that everything will be wonderful. Thus, as we end this chapter we plant a seed: Being honest about yourself means that you need to consider the possibility that the outcome of your journey will be a decision that you will *not* become a psychotherapist.

What Sharon says to her graduate classes is this: "Not everybody who applies to be in a counseling program should be in a counseling program. It just isn't the right niche for them." So, we'd like to give you a place to back out gracefully. There might be professions that better match with your ethical culture of origin. You may find that there aren't enough professional or personal motivations that can satisfy you as a therapist. The overlap between your personal motivations and values on the one hand and the values and motives expected of a therapist on the other may be small. You may find that there are other professions, or other professional activities, that will suit you better. It's OK to do so. It's OK to recognize that "this is not the profession for me." That's a good decision, an ethical decision.

By the way, this realization can also happen for people who have been working happily and effectively as psychotherapists for years. Life changes, people change, the profession changes. The journey is ongoing. Different priorities come up. Some therapists find a time in their careers when they say, "I need a change. This is not working for me any more."

If you decide that being a psychotherapist is not right for you, it doesn't necessarily mean that you become a salesperson, talk-show host, or professional wrestler. You may still become a counselor, social worker, or psychologist who does different activities, like assessment, consultation, or research.

Here's a related example from Sharon:

> My financial planner's associate has his doctorate in psychology. I found this information very interesting so I asked about the switch. He said that soon after his internship he decided that psychology was not what he wanted to do. He really likes working with people and he likes research and assessment, but he wanted a different context for these personal values and motivations. So when we're talking about my financial strategies, he goes back to the psychology literature to back up his points. What's intriguing to me is that he went through an entire doctoral program, he had the presence of mind and judgment to know it wasn't going to work for him, and he had the courage to make the switch.

We also decided to tell you that the two of us spend almost no time doing psychotherapy at this point in our careers. We write, consult, teach, administer, and train. We've both been psychotherapists at times in our lives and there may be times in the future when we do therapy again. At this point, helping you become an ethical therapist fulfills our values and motivations of helping students become ethically excellent therapists.

Part II

The Nuts and Bolts of Psychotherapy Ethics

4

The Ethical Culture of Psychotherapy

In our years of teaching and providing workshops in ethics to undergraduate, masters, and doctoral level students, both of us have had students get angry and discouraged. Much of the anger and frustration seemed to stem from students wanting us to just tell them "the answer" to an ethical dilemma. Early in our careers we were disconcerted by such reactions. Now we see them as a fairly typical, if not uncomfortable, part of ethical acculturation. The good news, of course, is that these students are learning such lessons as (a) not all ethical situations have clear answers; (b) it takes concentrated effort to resolve ethical dilemmas; and (c) the profession they are entering is a complex one.

Mitch remembers just recently a student in his ethics course who became discouraged with all the bad stuff that the class was discussing: violations of confidentiality, therapists having sex with clients, and other behaviors. The student began to think that she might not have the natural ability to become a therapist. As Mitch and the student discussed her feelings, it became clearer that she was having an acculturation crisis. The field of psychotherapy, she was learning, was much more than having clients come in with problems and therapists providing solutions. The skills involved in being a psychotherapist include, but are much more than, naturally occurring abilities and tendencies. In addition, the ethical dimensions of the profession and the skills necessary to appreciate those ethical dimensions are not usually intuitive.

Let's recap our progress thus far. In the first three chapters we've had you explore your motivations for becoming (and staying) a psychotherapist and your personal notions of right and wrong professional behavior. We've also encouraged you to take some time to explore your own self-care in times of personal and professional stress. We've even provided the opportunity for you to think about whether or not the profession is for you. In sum, we've encouraged you to take stock of your "culture of origin" using an ethical lens.

Now it is time to focus on the culture of psychotherapy to which you have been adapting. In this chapter, we focus on some of the major characteristics of this culture and ask you to reflect upon them. More specifically, we discuss the following aspects of the psychotherapy culture:

- guiding forces and Ethical Foundations for psychotherapists;
- aspects of psychotherapy that are different from other relationships;
- components of competence;
- precursors to good and bad therapist behaviors;
- ethical choice-making procedures.

If you are a seasoned therapist you will have much to reflect upon, including the changes you have seen in the professional culture over time. If you are a newcomer, however, you may be more able to identify the specific aspects of this new culture that are unexpected or that take some time to acclimatize to.

Ethical Foundations

You might think that therapists would or should simply be really nice people who have some good motivations and virtues. However, because of the complexity of psychotherapy and because of the high stakes and risk of harm, even the most virtuous people need more ethical guidance when they become professional therapists. This is where professional ethics come in.

Most mental health organizations have codes of professional ethics (e.g., National Association of Social Workers, 1999; American Association for Marriage and Family Therapy, 2001; American Psychological Association, 2002; American Counseling Association, 2005). The different codes of ethics vary to some degree, but we have boiled all these codes down to what we call the "Ethical Foundations for Psychotherapists." These are statements that highlight the ethical values in the culture of psychotherapy and act as basic guides for evaluating behavior:

1. **Do good** for clients and prospective clients. (This is also called *beneficence*.)
2. **Avoid doing harm** or exploiting clients. (This is also called *nonmaleficence*.)
3. Treat clients with **respect**. (This is also called *respect for autonomy*.)
4. Treat clients **fairly**. (This is also called *justice*.)
5. Become and remain **competent**.
6. Pursue your **interests without conflict**.
7. Maintain your **professional boundaries**.
8. Preserve **confidentiality**.
9. **Inform** clients of important information and get their **consent**.
10. Cultivate **virtues** including:
    - honesty
    - humility
    - diligence
    - prudence
    - integrity.

You can find links to more than 40 different professional ethics codes at http://kspope.com/ethcodes/index.php.

Notice three things about these Foundations. First, we've worded them all in as positive a way as possible. Second, they are not answers! Rather, they are guides. Third, they might conflict with each other in practice because of the complexity of the choices we make in psychotherapy.

Journal Entry: *Foundations*

Take a moment and reflect (in writing) on each one of the Ethical Foundations. Try to provide one example of something a therapist can do to follow or exemplify each Foundation, and one example of something a therapist can do that would violate the Foundation.

Psychotherapy Is a Unique Relationship

The psychotherapy relationship – perhaps more than any other professional relationship – is very potent and very fragile at the same time. By potent we mean that it can be a relationship that really enhances clients' lives and helps them grow. By fragile we mean that the relationship is delicate and must be handled with care; that is one of our major responsibilities as therapists.

Although psychotherapists are trained in a multitude of programs covering disciplines such as psychology, counseling, social work, family therapy, psychiatry, and a host of newer approaches, all therapeutic relationships share some essential features which we list now and then explore in some detail:

- The psychotherapy relationship includes professional care and concern – and it is not a "friendship."
- The therapy relationship is complex in terms of power.
- The general goal is for clients to be better after having experienced the relationship than before.
- Psychotherapists offer skill and expertise.
- The therapeutic relationship is built on trust.
- Therapists have ethical and legal responsibilities to clients.

The therapeutic relationship comprises professional care and concern We might be helpful in lots of relationships, yet the therapy relationship requires a unique kind of care and concern. As such, it is very different from friendship, a kind of relationship of which most of us have a lot of experience. Psychotherapists, in contrast to friends, must provide a different kind of human connection. For example, psychotherapists are there to work hard for and be there for clients – but not the other way around. The therapeutic relationship is asymmetrical; you cannot and should not expect the same kind of care and concern *from* your clients as you provide *to* your clients. (We talk more about this in chapter 5.)

Therapy represents a complex power relationship As psychotherapists we should be experts in human behavior and change, but we are not exclusively responsible for clients making changes or taking on new behaviors. The control over what happens in therapy, and to some extent the growth of clients, is shared between clients and us in our professional role – although in a complicated way. Here is what we mean: Clients have the power to decide whether to come, yet both therapists and clients share decision-making about the therapeutic goals and some of the general strategies. Therapists decide how to apply therapeutic techniques, yet clients make the decision whether to use or not use what they gained in session in their day-to-day lives. Both clients and psychotherapists decide whether therapy is working well enough to continue, yet clients ultimately decide whether their goals have been met and whether to continue with or to end therapy. (See chapter 9 for a fuller discussion of termination issues.)

The general goal is for clients to be better after having experienced the relationship than before   The relationship between clients and psychotherapists is meant to be functional and healthy, with clear boundaries and expectations. Through this healthy relationship, clients have the opportunity to see what good communication and respectful boundaries look and feel like. When therapists keep their personal needs out of the relationship and keep clients' needs first, clients will likely leave the relationship in better psychological/emotional health.

Psychotherapists offer skill and expertise   When clients purchase psychotherapy, they are really purchasing therapists' expertise and its appropriate use. It is this expertise that makes therapy a profession; consequently, psychotherapists have certain professional obligations. These obligations include knowing about how the therapeutic relationship works, understanding the dynamics of change and growth, knowing how to think about problems and their solutions, and recognizing the limits of their own professional competence.

The therapeutic relationship is built on trust   For good work to be done in therapy, clients need to trust their therapist in at least four ways:

1.   Clients need to trust that psychotherapists have the knowledge needed to help them make their lives better.
2.   Clients need to trust that psychotherapists are *using* skills and knowledge in ways that will help them.

3.   Clients need to trust that psychotherapists will be diligent and work hard with them in the therapy process.
4.   Clients need to trust that their well-being is the utmost priority in the therapy. As we explored in the previous chapter, this does not mean that therapists cannot meet any of their own needs in the profession. It does mean, however, that getting these needs met should *not* come at the expense of clients' well-being and goal attainment.

Therapists have ethical and legal responsibilities   Ethical principles and values underlie every aspect of psychotherapy. For example, the principle of beneficence that constitutes our Foundation #1 – doing good – justifies the existence of the entire psychotherapy profession. It also means doing an excellent job by keeping in mind why the relationship is there in the first place. Ethics provides a positive base for our work that can help us work toward ethical excellence as well as avoid problems and complaints.

In addition to ethical responsibilities, therapists have legal responsibilities to clients. Because the therapeutic relationship is fragile and therapists can exploit and harm clients, many of the professions that practice psychotherapy are regulated by states and provinces. Regulations identify therapists' obligations and clarify legal protections for clients. For example, the psychotherapy relationship may be recognized legally as a privileged relationship (see chapter 6) similar to the doctor–patient relationship.

As a psychotherapist you might see ethics codes and laws as constraints – long lists of prohibited behaviors and the punishments involved. However, good work happens when we are working from the lens of "wanting to do the best for the client" (a "positive" principle) rather than from the lens of "this is a hassle, but I don't want to get into trouble" (a "constraint" principle).

Competence: What It Is and What It Isn't

Competence is not the same as licensure, academic degrees, credentials, attendance at workshops, authored books, or a nice office. Any and all of these suggest or might suggest some knowledge and some skill level but they say nothing about ability, diligence, humility or wisdom. In addition, competence is not simply the absence of harm (Foundation #2).

From the more traditional lens of ethics, we as psychotherapists want the client to receive some level of benefit from our work together. From the positive ethics and ethical excellence lens, we really want to shoot for the ethical ceiling – we want to do everything on our end of the professional relationship to help the client. We aren't talking perfection here or working harder than the client. What we are talking about is keeping track of or monitoring ourselves on five components of competence and assessing where we are on the competence continuum (Koocher, 1979). Between the two of them, Kitchener (2000) and Welfel (2006) identify four of the five components: knowledge of the literature; skill (technical and clinical) to act on that knowledge; ability (both emotional and physical) to effectively work with the client; and diligence or "going the extra mile" and consistently making sure the client's well-being is our top priority. We add a fifth component, which is drawing upon the virtues of humility and wisdom. We need to know when we have hit our limit or boundary of expertise and to recognize that we can't work with every client.

Now you might be thinking, "So, how do I know if and when I am competent? And it sounds like competence or my level of competence can change. Is that right?" These are really good questions and, yes, competence can fluctuate – even on a daily basis (Welfel, 2006). To help you answer these questions, we've developed the following questions for you to ask yourself.

Questions about the knowledge component:
- What does the current literature say about my clients and their issues?
- How would I explain my current working knowledge to my best clinical supervisor?

Questions about the skill component:
- In keeping up with the literature, what new skills am I employing effectively?
- How do I know that I am implementing these skills effectively? What am I using to assess my effectiveness?

Questions about the ability component:
- How am I taking care of my own emotional state so that I am able to really be there for my clients?
- How am I taking care of myself physically so that I am in good health?

Questions about the diligence component:
- How am I doing with keeping my clients' needs at the top of the priority list?
- What is my most recent example of "going the extra mile" in my psychotherapy practice?

Questions about the virtue component:
- What are the boundaries of my expertise?
- How have I used supervision, consultation, or my own personal therapy lately to assess my current level of effectiveness as a psychotherapist?

Multicultural Competence

Part of the notion of competence (Foundation #5) is competence with people from a variety of cultural backgrounds. Sue and Sue (2003) define multicultural competence as having three dimensions: (a) being aware of your own values, beliefs, biases, and notions about human-kind and its nature; (b) having a general understanding or knowledge of worldviews different from your own but without negative judgment toward these other worldviews; and (c) having the skills and know-ledge to use psychotherapy interventions that are fitting with diverse clients. We would add a fourth dimension to this list which is the fol-lowing: (d) coming to know your own points of privilege so that you can hear another's experience of being invisible, devalued, disrespected because of their gender, skin color, age, partner choice, economic status, being differently abled, choice of spirituality, etc. Having these four dimensions in place would translate into competence to work with individuals different from ourselves. As our world is becoming more and more culturally diverse, it means that multicultural competence is no longer a luxury of psychotherapists but a necessity of ethical practice.

Now you may be thinking, "Wait a minute! How can I be multicul-turally competent in my practice? What if there are some groups that I don't know about? What if there are some worldviews I disagree with? What if ...?" These are great questions and they suggest your desire to be transparent. It is easier in the short run to try and ignore the unfamil-iar and avoid areas of disagreement. We are glad you're not doing either of these.

Here is what we say to our students who have asked these questions: First, give yourself some growing room. None of us can be a multicultural expert with all cultures. We can, however, be lifelong learners and willing to access experience, training, and consultation to gain multicultural competence. Second, not everyone who wants or asks to work with you will be someone you can serve. In this sense, multicultural competence is similar to other types of competence. As a psychotherapist you will be clear about your limits of competence and it would be unethical for you to go beyond those limits. This is also true about differing worldviews. You may not be able to work competently with someone whose worldview is very different from yours. The issue here should be one of different perspectives without disrespect.

Journal Entry: *My Current Location on the Road to Multicultural Competence*

Make a list of three cultures you feel you know a lot about. Write a couple of sentences after each culture explaining how you know about the culture. Then make a list of three cultures you know nothing or very little about, with a couple sentences for each one including a brief statement about your attitudes toward these cultures and a statement of how interested you are in gaining some understanding. (Allow yourself the luxury of being honest.)

Now, on a scale from 1 to 5, with 1 being "not at all descriptive of me" and 5 being "perfectly descriptive of me," rate each of the following thoughts and how much they apply to you at this moment:

_____I don't need any more information on other cultures than I have now.

_____I can't work with anybody about whose culture I am not perfectly expert.

_____I know I have cultural weak spots. I am a little anxious about this but want to develop a strategy to (a) overcome them and/or (b) lessen their impact.

This activity gives you some information about your acculturation journey as it relates to multicultural competence. If you identified with the first statement, "I don't need any more information on other cultures than I have now," you might be adopting a separation strategy. If you identified with the second statement, "I can't work with anybody about whose culture I am not perfectly expert," you might be using an assimilation strategy. If the third statement reflects more of your "current location" then you might be using an integration strategy.

Journal Entry: *Professional Behaviors*

Psychotherapy can be defined by appropriate professional behaviors – those that are consistent with the Ethical Foundations and that most clients expect of psychotherapists.

Part 1   Make a list of behaviors that might occur in (a) psychotherapy relationships, and (b) friendships.

Part 2   Identify which behaviors overlap between (a) and (b), and which behaviors should only occur in therapy relationships or only in friendships.

Part 3   Identify the Ethical Foundations that justify your placement of each of the behaviors in your lists.

Precursors to Good and Bad Therapist Behaviors: Green and Red Flags

It is one thing to understand on a theoretical level that ethical psychotherapists will be "respectful," or that unethical psychotherapists will "exploit" clients; but what do respect and exploitation look like in practice? What indicators might there be in our everyday behaviors as therapists that suggest we are on the right (or wrong) track? In this section we look at good and bad behavior and do this by introducing the concept of green flags and red flags.

What Are Green Flags and Red Flags?

When people asked us several years ago what we were working on we said something like, "We're writing a book to help psychotherapists stop and really think about their behavioral choices with clients." We were amazed at how many people responded to this news with stories of their own experiences with psychotherapists. Here's one of the stories where we think the psychotherapist who did really good work.

> I had a friend refer me to his therapist. Man, I was in a world of hurt. Well, I made the call and this therapist was great. I mean it was a safe place for me to share my life story and not feel judged. I remember one time when I really just wanted her to tell me what I should do in a relationship, but she didn't. At the time I felt really frustrated, but as we talked I realized how she was allowing me to take responsibility for myself and not take the easy way out. Looking back, I really like how she helped me figure out what therapy was all about, and what I wanted and needed in a relationship.

We see this as a great example of ethical work. First, the psychotherapist did a good job of respecting the client's autonomy (Foundation #3) by encouraging him to arrive at his own answers. Second, our friend says he felt safe and not judged by the therapist. From our view, this therapist was doing good, manifesting beneficence (Foundation #1). We congratulated our friend for finding an ethical psychotherapist who demonstrates some of the green flags we'll share a little later.

On the other hand, we had friends tell us stories about psychotherapists whose behaviors were odd or dubious. Here is one example that demonstrates red flags:

> You know, I went to a therapist once, and it only lasted one session. I wanted to get over some test anxiety – I learned things well in class, but when I took tests, I couldn't do well. So I went to

this therapist, and for a lot of the session he talked about things like, oh, getting a lucky pencil – the one I used when I studied and got practice questions right. He said this'd give me confidence. And then, about 45 minutes into the session, he told me I really should stop at a lingerie store on my way home and get a really sexy pair of panties and wear those to the test to make me feel sexy and confident. It kind of creeped me out. I shot out of there and never went back.

Behaviors that Indicate Green Flags

Therapists who are demonstrating ethical or good behaviors are consistently meeting many if not all of the Ethical Foundations. For example, good therapists are humble (Foundation #10), and they are realistic about what they can reasonably expect to accomplish. They are diligent about providing good and clear information (Foundation #9) to clients so that clients will make better decisions (Foundation #1). Therapists behaving ethically will not guarantee success; however, they will guarantee that they are trying really hard to help. Being guarded in this way is also respectful of clients (Foundation #3). Please note that we used the words "consistently meeting" rather than "perfectly meeting" the Ethical Foundations. None of us is perfect; however, we need to take our responsibility for ethical practice to heart. Kitchener (2000) says it this way:

> Issues of responsibility are some of the most difficult with which to deal in a profession like psychology (counseling) because our work affects other humans. At the same time, we cannot be held to a superhuman standard that never allows for an error in judgment … It is not a standard of perfection. At the same time, we must aspire to provide the most effective services … of which we are capable. (p. 184)

Green flags are indicators that the therapist has good judgment, a good attitude, and a professional approach. The following is a list of green flags:

Amicable Advice about Alternatives. Therapists will help clients find the best therapy for them, rather than talking them into the therapists' own services.

Responsible Referrals. Therapists will make suggestions about who might be able to provide help for clients, especially when therapy is not working.

Informative Information. Therapists provide useful information about therapy and respond to client questions in understandable language.

Clear Consent. Therapists explicitly seek consent to treatment and revisit this consent at various points in the therapy (for example, when goals change).

Good Goals. After the first few sessions (although it could be sooner), therapists and clients need to be clear about therapy goals.

Guarded Guarantees. Therapists are humble and realistic about their work and they do not guarantee success. The only guarantee they do make is to work hard to help.

Beneficial Boundary Bolstering. Therapists will let clients know about boundaries and enforce those boundaries even where clients plead for an exception.

Effective Ethical Explanations. Therapists will explain the decisions they make.

Ethical Explorations. Therapists will ask clients to explore actions and feelings, even when this is uncomfortable. "You're interested in aspects of my private life. I wonder where that might be coming from."

Requests for Written Releases. Therapists request written permission to share information about clients with appropriate professionals, such as physicians or attorneys.

Ethical Endings. Therapists recognize when therapy needs to end (clients have accomplished their goals, or therapy is not being effective), and they facilitate good closure.

Green Flag: *Guarded Guarantees*

Let us explore the following vignette:

> Della had calmed down considerably from the beginning of her first session with Dr Hawkins. But she was still quite anxious. "I'm gonna be OK, aren't I, Doc?"
>
> Dr Hawkins wanted to be as supportive as he could. "Della, you've done a good thing by coming into therapy. You've made a good start today. I'll be happy to see you next week."

"But Doctor, you can make me feel better, can't you?"

"I can work with you to try."

"But I need a guaranTEE!!" said Della, knowing as she said it that she wasn't going to get it.

"I can tell you're very upset," replied Dr Hawkins evenly. "You'd really like to know that the hard work you're about to put in will pay off. And for most clients, it does. But I can't guarantee any particular result. All I can do is guarantee that I'll work as hard as I can with you. And if we find, after a while, that therapy isn't going the way you'd like, I'll be happy to give you some names of other therapists who might be more helpful."

Part 1   To begin your exploration, put yourself in the position of Della, the client:

- How do you feel when Dr Hawkins responds the way he does?
- Imagine Dr Hawkins is different from you – maybe a different ethnic background, different religion, different sexual orientation, different gender, and/or different age, or having a physical disability. Do your reactions change under these different conditions?

Part 2   Imagine other professional situations in which you have been a client (e.g., seeing a physician, accountant, or auto mechanic, or hiring a band for a wedding, or purchasing a riding lawnmower):

- What kinds of guarantees would you expect from those professionals?
- How are these expectations similar to or different from your expectations of Dr Hawkins?

Part 3   Put yourself in the position of Dr Hawkins:

- How did you feel when Della demanded a guarantee? Threatened? Confused? Angry? Powerful? Surprised?
- How would you have responded? What acculturation strategy might your response have reflected?
- Imagine that Della is different from you – maybe a different ethnic background, different religion, different sexual orientation, different gender, and/or different age, or having a physical disability. Do your reactions change under these different conditions?

- How else could you have demonstrated respect for Della and still not provided an inappropriate guarantee? What might be some good integration strategies?
- How would your response have been different if Della …
  - was just a casual friend of yours asking for advice?
  - was a neighbor asking you to keep the noise down at your house?

Behaviors that Indicate Red Flags

Remember the story from one of our friends – the one about her therapist suggesting that she (our friend) buy and wear a "sexy pair of panties" to boost her confidence for taking a test? During this conversation with our friend, we talked about the fact that this suggestion might have been an innocent comment and not a sexual overture. Dealing with sex in therapy is just like dealing with money, marriage, anxiety, depression, and other aspects of human existence. But we also agreed that making this particular comment, innocent or not, showed extremely poor judgment on the part of the therapist. We thought our friend was smart to leave that office and not go back. If the psychotherapist was not a sexual pervert, he was probably showing a preview of more bad choices (aka red flags) to come.

Sexual remarks made out of context, or undue focus on sex, is one of the easiest precursors or red flags to spot. But there are lots of other warning signs that are smaller, more subtle, and harder to detect. At a minimum, red flags are indicators of poor judgment. They are certainly signs that therapists may not be taking their professional responsibilities as seriously as they should. We are not saying that each of these red flags is, in itself, unethical or unprofessional behavior. We are saying, however, that the red flags may at least be precursors to more serious problems. The following is a list of red flags:

Everybody's Everything. Therapists convey, directly or indirectly, that they can handle every problem, often because of what good therapists they are. This shows a naive and simplistic attitude toward complex phenomena (human emotion and behavior). This red flag could also be called Lacking Clarity on the Limits of Competence.

Dissing the Different. Therapists are overly disparaging of other therapists or other approaches.

Excessive Enthusiasm for Exclusive Enterprises. Therapists will try to sell one type of therapy, or one answer to all problems, rather than appreciating that there are lots of ways to solve problems. For example, "What you need is hypnosis! It works wonders for all my clients, and for me."

Defensive Declarations. Therapists will "pull rank" when challenged, rather than address clients' concerns. For example, "You're not supposed to ask me that question. I'm the therapist here."

Logistical Laxity. This refers to evidence of sloppiness. Forgetting appointments, not having the right forms available, not keeping adequate records – all indicate that for some reason therapists are not taking care of business.

Exciting Exceptions Equal Excruciating Effects. Therapists make exceptions to their usual policies. This behavior is especially problematic when they advertise that they are doing so. "I wouldn't do this with my other clients, but …"

Shared Secrets Seem Suspicious. Therapists are secretive about certain activities in therapy. "This'll be just our little secret."

Compromised Confidentiality. Therapists will violate client privacy and confidentiality by sharing information with others. For example, therapists leave files and correspondence on the desk with clients' names within the field of vision of anyone who might come into their office.

Porous Privacy. Therapists share information about one client with another client. This can be on a continuum: The most problematic is a full disclosure, with names and/or other identifying information about some experience of clients. This conduct can also take the form of bragging, with therapists telling stories about their triumphs. It can be more subtle, like simply illustrating a point with an example with too much detail.

Intimations of Inappropriate Intimacy. Therapists blur boundaries between a professional and personal relationship.

Invidious Invitations. Therapists invite clients to functions or events that are not part of therapy.

Reprehensible Rationalizations. Therapists offer explanations to clients for behaving unethically that may sound good but are only rationalizations for breaking the rules. The simplest and perhaps most dangerous: "Just this once."

Spiritual Selling. Discussing spiritual or religious issues in therapy may be just fine if it is related to clients' goals. But it is *not* a good sign when therapists force their spiritual perspective on clients or invite clients to their place of worship.

Sideline Solicitations. Therapists offer a service or product for sale that is not part of therapy. For example, they offer to do clients' taxes, or to sell clients their old CD player.

Counterproductive Curiosity about Clients. Therapy, by its very nature, deals with very personal experiences and issues. When therapists get too interested in hearing interesting details that are not therapeutically relevant, they are letting their own interests (prurient or otherwise) get in the way.

We anticipate at least two possible reactions from you as you read through the list of red flags and the red flag stories throughout the rest of the book. Your first reaction might be, "No therapist would do anything that extreme/stupid/unethical." Some of these stories are more extreme than others, but we want you to know that they are all based on actual cases we are familiar with – although we've disguised identities and facts to preserve privacy.

The second reaction you might have is, "*I* would never do anything like that!" We encourage you to bear in mind that good people can and do end up doing unethical things. Unethical behaviors are not restricted to a certain class or type of psychotherapist. We are human, with complex motivations, and psychotherapy is a complex, unique, powerful, and fragile process. Consequently, we are all capable of unethical behaviors. You will get more out of these stories by considering the conditions or motivations under which you would act similarly rather than creating distance between you and the therapists depicted.

Red Flag: *Logistical Laxity*

Consider the following story:

> Sarah paced up and down the long, thin hallway in the office building. Dr Horne's office was at the far end of the hallway, away

from the elevators, so Sarah would not miss spotting Dr Horne. It was already 8:25, and they had an 8:00 appointment. Sarah was happy that Dr Horne made this early appointment (rather than the usual 8:30) so she could make it to a work meeting on time, but now she felt like there might not be any session at all. She tried to remember what they said in college about how long students had to wait for what kind of professor.

At the stroke of 8:30, Dr Horne came rushing out of the elevator, her face hardly visible behind a large purse, a leather brief case, a laptop case, several paperback books, and a tote bag from the local public radio station. Even while carrying all that, Dr Horne was jiggling her key ring loudly, trying to lay her finger on her office keys. "Good morning!" she said brightly.

Sarah said, "Uh, we were scheduled for 8:00."

"Oh, were we? I must have forgotten to check my book. Don't we usually meet at 8:30?"

"Yes, but we changed it last time, remember?"

"Oh yes," Dr Horne responded. "But we can go a few minutes later. My next client won't mind."

That's really not the point, thought Sarah. She felt let down when she thought Dr Horne wasn't going to show at all. And besides, she was wanting to do some heavy work. Now it was hard for her to "gear up" again to have a good session. Should she just leave? Would Dr Horne charge her?

Here are some questions to consider:

- What's it like to be "stood up" in this way? How does it make you feel?
- Which of the Ethical Foundations might Dr Horne have violated?
- How serious would you judge the violations to be? For example, how much harm was done?
- What virtues might Dr Horne need to cultivate?
- How often are you late for appointments?
- What other behaviors might you exhibit that would be included in "logistical laxity"? Sloppy record-keeping? Forgetfulness? How do they influence the relationships you are in? How might they influence your therapy relationships? What acculturation strategies might be reflected in logistical laxity? What strategies might be good alternatives?

Journal Entry: *Ethics Autobiography, Part 2*

In chapter 1 you started your ethics autobiography by discussing your ethics of origin, your notions of right and wrong that you brought with you into the profession. In this part of the Ethics Autobiography, we ask you to explore your professional culture.

If you are a student or a new professional, we encourage you to start here with these questions. If you are a practicing psychotherapist, you can focus on your initial training as you answer these questions or drop down to the next set of questions.

- What have you learned about the culture of psychotherapy that you did not expect?
- What have you learned about or been asked to do that has been counterintuitive, surprising, or puzzling?

This will get you started focusing on your acculturation tasks. If you find a lot that has been counterintuitive, you may be facing acculturation stress or crises – large disconnects between your goals/motivations/values and your ability to meet those goals as a psycho-therapist.

Here are some other questions to consider:

- What parts of your new profession fit easily into who you are and which parts do not (did not) seem like such a good fit?
- How have your personal relationships changed as a result of becoming a psychotherapist?

If you have been in the profession long enough, take a few minutes to answer these questions:

- How has the profession changed since you entered it?
- How have you changed since you first became a therapist?
- As you look back, what aspects of your professional development may have been an interaction between your personal changes and changes in the profession?

One final question:

- What personal and professional changes might you need to deal with in the next few years (e.g., divorce, retirement, empirically supported treatments, the rise of coaching)?

Ethical Choice Process

Virtually all ethics books include decision-making procedures (Cottone & Claus, 2000). Cottone, Tarvydas, and Claus (2007) provide an overview of ethical decision-making models in the psychology and counseling fields. What we have seen is that most models focus on the need to take the following steps:

- identify the problem;
- develop and analyze alternatives using relevant codes, guidelines, laws, regulations, policies;
- consult with other professionals;
- choose, implement, and evaluate the decision.

Many books refer to this as an *ethical decision-making* model or procedure. Anderson, Wagoner, and Moore (2006) chose to use the term *ethical choice process* instead. The word *choice* emphasizes the active process of implementing ethical decisions over the cognitive exercise of identifying the issues and analyzing the codes and principles. The word *process* suggests the fluid, nonlinear, and interactive nature of the model. In some ways it is similar to a feedback loop. New information at any one step can impact the other steps along the way.

As we have seen, making ethical choices involves and is influenced by several factors. These factors include (a) our values and the match between our values and those of the profession; (b) our personal character or virtues; (c) moral reasoning; (d) our professional training in ethics; and (e) our professional ethical identity that has developed through acculturation to the profession.

The following ethical choice-making process expands on the steps outlined above. It is adapted from a previous work by Anderson and colleagues (2006), and includes steps and questions from a multitude of other sources. The centerpiece of the model draws upon Rest's four components of moral behavior. To highlight each of the components and illuminate the process within each one, we present representative questions for therapists to consider. These questions tap into psychotherapists' thinking, motivations, values, needs, and possible conflicts of interest. In addition, the questions show the importance of perspective-taking and including client input at appropriate times. Remember also that Rest (1994) does not describe these components as occurring in a linear or sequential fashion; his contention is that each component has to occur for moral behavior to be the outcome.

Component 1 – ethical sensitivity These questions encourage psychotherapists to develop sensitivity to the issues at hand and how alternative choices will affect others positively and negatively:

- What strikes you as strange or makes you uncomfortable?
- What demands your attention?
- Who is involved in this situation?
- What makes you think, "Uh-oh, this doesn't feel right"?
- What makes you think, "Yes, this feels good or right"?
- What are the issues related to diversity? To differences between my client and me? To oppression or discrimination?
- How does my point of privilege affect my sensitivity to this issue?
- How does my value set affect my sensitivity to this issue?
- What new value or values do I need to cultivate?

Component 2 – formulating an ethical plan These questions prompt psychotherapists to evaluate what they know about the scenario and how the code speaks to the ethical problem. It also encourages psychotherapists to view the issue from the client's perspective.

- What do I know about the situation? What are the facts of the case?
- What else do I need to know?
- What does the ethical code have to say about this situation?
- What ethical standards conflict in this situation?

- What are the legal issues involved?
- With whom should I consult?
- What do I need to explain or share with the client about the ethical issue?
- If I were the client, what would I hope my psychotherapist would share with me?
- If I were the client, what would I hope my psychotherapist would do?
- From what I know right now, what choices would be the most positive and closest to an integration strategy?

Component 3 – ethical motivation and competing values   These questions call for psychotherapists to identify conflicts of interest and their personal motivations and values that are competing with professional values:

- What are my personal values and motivations in this situation?
- What are my professional obligations in this situation?
- Is there a match between the two or is there a conflict?
- If I am experiencing acculturation stress, which acculturation strategy am I leaning toward implementing and why?
- If there is a conflict between my personal values and professional values, can I express my values and motivation in a different way?
- If there is a conflict, how can I reorganize or reprioritize my personal values?
- With whom might I consult to see the conflicts as clearly as possible?
- What core values (personal and professional) are being stretched?
- What core values (personal and professional) are being strengthened?
- How does my client win or lose, depending on the course of action?

Component 4 – ethical follow-through   These questions prompt implementation of the choice:

- To whom or what (e.g., the law) must I be accountable? To whom do I want to be accountable?

- Who in my professional circles can encourage or support me to do the right thing?
- What personal and professional values do I need to draw upon?
- What did I say in my ethics autobiography that would help me at this point in time?
- As I implement this choice, what do I need to let the client know?

Conclusion

In Part I, we introduced you to your acculturation task and invited you to become more aware of your ethical background and your motivations for entering the field. In this chapter we presented, in broad terms, the principles and values that characterize the profession of psychotherapy and an ethical choice-making process. Thus, the basic foundations of acculturation are now in place.

Now it is time to explore (or re-explore) the culture of psychotherapy in enough detail to give you a sense of how your acculturation is progressing. In the next chapters in Part II we go more deeply into the ethical traditions and themes of psychotherapy, including chapters on boundaries, confidentiality, informed consent, supervision and termination. As you work through these chapters it will be a good idea to keep with you the journal entries and exercises you have done thus far. Maintaining your awareness of your own backgrounds, motivations, and goals, along with the ethical foundations of psychotherapy, will help you avoid moving too far into the strategies of assimilation, separation, or marginalization, and will keep your eyes on *your own* path toward excellence.

5

"I Can't Believe It's Not Therapy!"
Boundaries of the Psychotherapy Relationship

Food for Thought: *Boundaries*

> Anita has been seeing her therapist, Dr Bolden, for several months. Toward the end of a recent session, Dr Bolden begins sharing little tidbits about his own relationships. His wife, he tells Anita, is frequently out of town. He goes on to say that their interests, which were similar at one time, are now very different and their sexual intimacy is almost nonexistent. Anita feels a little funny about what Dr Bolden is saying, but she feels like he must trust her a lot to share such intimate details. At the next session, Dr Bolden compliments Anita on the progress she's made as he literally pats her on the back. This makes Anita feel really good. As he continues to keep his hand on Anita's shoulder, Dr Bolden suggests as a kind of celebration, that they meet for their next session at a quaint little restaurant near the office. Feeling only a little uncomfortable but very pleased with praise by a therapist, Anita accepts the invitation. At the restaurant, Dr Bolden makes a sexual advance, which Anita angrily rebuffs. After only a few more sessions, Anita's condition worsens.

Given what you read in the last chapter, what aspects of Dr Bolden's behavior cause you concern? What red flags do you see? At what point did you feel that Dr Bolden's behavior was no longer appropriate? What Foundations might he be violating? What virtues might he not have enough, or too much, of? What might you speculate about the acculturation strategies he is using?

So far you've explored your ethical culture of origin and you've examined the general principles and values that characterize the culture of psychotherapy. In short, you've laid the foundations for the acculturation process into the profession of psychotherapy, and you've started your journey. Now you are ready to hone your acculturation skills by applying them to a series of key ethical issues.

Because psychotherapy is done behind closed doors, misconceptions abound concerning what is and what is not psychotherapy. TV and movies routinely portray therapists and clients behaving and interacting in ways that go beyond the therapy relationship – for example, having romantic encounters. In addition, your friends might mention that they had a therapy session at a coffee shop, or that their therapists talked a lot about their own troubles, not just the clients'. These interactions make it sound like some of your friends and their therapists are engaged in a friendship, not therapy. You might be wondering – was that OK or did the therapist do something wrong?

In the following pages we will highlight several key points about the therapy relationship that relate to professional boundaries. We will start with some foundational information about boundaries and move to more specific discussions about types of boundary crossings and boundary violations, multiple role relationships, and other appropriate and inappropriate boundaries between therapists and clients.

Boundaries: What They Are and Why They Are So Important

Having to consider boundaries may initially feel counterintuitive. In real life, we all have multiple roles in our relationships with other people. Where one relationship ends and the other begins is not clear – nor does it always need to be. For example, we buy insurance from our friends, we invite our neighbors to come with us to lectures at the public library, and we play bridge with the parents of our children's friends. The culture of psychotherapy, however, necessitates a much more defined and constrained professional role. Within this role is an expected set of behaviors which reflect the Ethical Foundations (p. 73). These behaviors include:

- listening actively to clients (Foundations #1 and #5);
- treating clients with respect (Foundation #3), especially when we are confronting them;
- telling clients when we think we are no longer effective in our work with them (Foundations #1 and #2).

The line between what is part of the role as psychotherapist and what is not is called a *professional boundary* (Gutheil & Gabbard, 1993). In other words, it is the line between the therapy relationship and some other type of relationship with the client. Crossing or violating a professional boundary can compromise the goals and focus of the professional relationship.

There is certainly a continuum of perspectives regarding what is right, good, or beneficial and what is wrong, bad, or harmful when it comes to boundaries. Of course, there are some boundaries that all ethical psychotherapists would say should not be crossed (e.g., sexual relationships between therapists and clients), but other boundaries or relationships are matters of ongoing debate. We have our own perspective and will encourage you to explore your stance on these issues.

Red Flags: *Invidious Invitations and Reprehensible Rationalizations*

> In the third session with Dr Vaughan, Lena finds herself being asked to lunch by her therapist! Lena knows this isn't a recognized part of therapy and she's heard that it's not really a good idea ... But she's hungry! And Dr Vaughan is making a good case for lunch being very convenient. "Look, we're both hungry; I know I missed my lunch. How about if we walk down to the coffee shop on the corner for our session – that way we'll be able to talk without being so edgy."

In reading the story above both the client and the psychotherapist, Dr Vaughan, are suggesting that they accomplish two goals simultaneously: productive therapy time and eating. Think through the following questions:

- If you are the client, Lena, what is your initial reaction? What are you feeling? What do you think of the suggestion?
- Based on your initial reaction, what or how would you respond to Dr Vaughan's suggestion?
- Put yourself in Dr Vaughan's position. Besides being hungry and wanting to get lunch, what are other possible motivations behind your request or suggestion?
- If you were a supervisor of Dr Vaughan's and she shared this situation with you, how would you respond to her? What would your motivations be for your response?
- What acculturation strategy might be reflected in Dr Vaughan's behavior? What other behaviors would you encourage her to consider as she works toward integration?
- What if Dr Vaughan suggested a session at a colleague's office that's closer to her home? A park? A study room at a public library?

Boundary Crossings and Violations

Gutheil and Gabbard (1993) make the distinction between boundary *crossings* and boundary *violations*. Boundary crossings refer to minor and momentary slips from the role of therapist to another role. For example, in some cultures clients may expect psychotherapists in the community to participate in weddings or memorial services and then return to their original role. In fact, the participation in the wedding or service may be an issue for discussion in therapy before and after the event.

Other boundary crossings may be more subtle and avoidable and lead down the slippery slope to boundary *violations*. Violations are serious breaches of boundaries that are potentially harmful to the therapeutic relationship and exploitative of clients (Gutheil & Gabbard, 1993). Any behavior that brings a nontherapeutic intimacy or closeness into the relationship is a boundary violation.

Sometimes it is hard to tell if a particular behavior is a boundary crossing or violation. For example, you decide to offer a client a ride home because their car won't start or you routinely let the therapy time go past the allotted time for the session. Determining whether these behaviors are crossings or violations may seem like an intellectual exercise. Reflecting on the difference, however, *before* engaging in the behaviors, can help you make better decisions. One way you can tell whether a boundary violation is the issue is to consider whether you are making an exception to a professional or ethical policy that you have. Here's a scenario for you to consider.

Red Flag: *Exciting Exceptions Equal Excruciating Effects*

Jeanne, who had been laid off from her office manager job at age 52, gets the name of a "cute" therapist from a friend of hers who met him when she took skiing lessons from him last winter. The therapist, Dr Parker, prides himself on being able to relate especially well to women who are suffering from loneliness and depression. He tells Jeanne that she doesn't have to call him Doctor, and, interestingly enough, he never really tells her what his doctorate is in or where it's from.

During the second session, Jeanne is discussing her financial problems when Dr Parker interrupts her to say, "Listen, I know I shouldn't do this, but how would you like to be my secretary for just a few weeks? I'm writing a book and could use some extra help."

Jeanne has never been in therapy, but she has this funny feeling inside and asks tentatively, "Is that OK, I mean, hiring a client of yours?"

"Well, technically," Dr Parker says, "it's not really considered a good thing. But we're both mature people, and I'm sure we can handle the issues that may come up." Even as she struggles not to, Jeanne finds herself feeling flattered and special. And spending "extra" time with Dr Parker might help her feel less lonely.

Think about the motivations of both Dr Parker and Jeanne. Dr Parker might be thinking he is just crossing a boundary and there's no potential for harm. What do you think? How would you encourage Dr Parker to move toward an integration strategy? What virtues might he want to develop?

Sometimes we might be tempted to justify a behavior or protest too hard to make it feel more acceptable. Such temptations are good examples of acculturation stress. The justification or protesting may be evidence of a separation or marginalization strategy. This doesn't make the behavior more acceptable or right. In fact, the professional codes exist for just these situations.

Journal Entry: *When Does a Boundary Crossing Become a Boundary Violation?*

Think about your own possible temptations with clients. Write down 4–5 things you might do or say with clients that are not really part of therapy. For each one, ask yourself these questions to help determine when a boundary crossing becomes a violation:

- What is the potential harm (e.g., of giving a client a ride home, loaning a client $30 to pay the phone bill, etc.)? The answer to this question may not be so easy to figure out and may hinge on several other factors:
  - What is the client's type and degree of emotional or psychological disturbance?
  - What impact might there be of the gender, cultural backgrounds, and ages of both you and the client?
  - What might the client expect in this situation? What are their motivations?
  - What are your motivations for crossing this boundary?
  - What motivations might be perceived or inferred by others, such as members of the client's family, close colleagues of yours, and ethics committee members?

- Is the behavior temporary or likely to be ongoing?
- What is your reaction the second time a client asks for a ride home, a small loan, or a coffee between sessions?
- Does the behavior represent a move toward a permanent (rather than temporary) realignment of the roles between you and your client?
- What alternatives exist that would be therapeutic, respectful, and less of a crossing?

Sometimes the type or degree of a behavior may be signs of impending problems. For example, too much or the wrong kind of (a) giving advice, (b) your own self-disclosure, and (c) touching are all boundary crossings and can lead to boundary violations. Let's take a look at each of these in more detail.

Giving Advice

How do you know when you are giving too much advice, the wrong kind of advice, or should even be giving advice at all? Giving advice is a very controversial issue and therapists' practices vary widely, based on their theoretical orientation and their personalities.

Food for Thought: *Acculturating to Giving Advice*

Think of your cultures of origin – family relationships, friendships, previous job situations, and others.

- How much specific advice do you generally give in these relationships?
- What role does advice play in these relationships?
- What kinds of advice do you find most and least helpful?

- What types of acculturation strategies might you be tempted to use regarding giving advice?
- How might you think about moving toward integration?

The easiest red flag to notice may simply be that you are giving too much advice, especially early in therapy. Too much advice may be a sign of a separation strategy: you are talking to clients as if they were friends. It may show disrespect (Foundation #3) by communicating that you know more than clients do about their own lives. It may also be flat-out incompetent (Foundation #5).

One indicator of incompetent advice is when you find that you are offering lots of advice on the basis of relatively little information. Here, you might want to stop and ask yourself, "Am I trying to impress the client more than trying to help? Am I more willing to give advice because I find this client attractive in some way? Am I trying to get clients to be like me or my vision of them rather than becoming more like themselves?"

On the other hand, as a psychotherapist you can be using an assimilation strategy by giving too little advice. When this happens, you may be trying to create a relationship in which clients can develop their own answers. The good news about this approach is that it is very respectful of clients' abilities to think, work, and grow. It maintains very clear boundaries and avoids the situation in which you give clients bad advice. The bad news is that it can be frustrating for clients when you will not share any opinions at all.

How much advice is one dimension to consider; another dimension is the kind of advice. It may be useful to think about two major kinds of advice, which we call *process* advice and *substantive* advice.

- Process advice consists of suggestions for how to go about solving problems, or how to make the most of therapy.
- Substantive advice consists of suggestions for specific solutions to the problems, or for how to live.

We think it is more justifiable for therapists to give process advice than substantive advice. For example, we believe advice on how to think through a career decision (process) is more acceptable than advice on whether to take the job (substantive). On the whole, we think it is better for therapists to err in the direction of giving too little advice rather than seeing it as just part of the usual routine.

Therapist Self-disclosure

Self-disclosure by the psychotherapist can be prompted in various ways. We may feel like sharing a personal story or issue which might help clients. Another common prompt for self-disclosure is when clients ask us personal questions. It is natural for our clients to want to know about us as people (Braaten, Otto, & Handelsman, 1993; Braaten & Handelsman, 1997). It can even feel good, perhaps flattering, to have a client curious about us and who we are.

How to handle the issue of self-disclosure is a key acculturation task. On one side of this issue are arguments that center around the virtues of honesty and openness. You may feel like part of establishing a good working relationship is (a) being honest with a client, and (b) being open about who you are. For sure, some personal questions from clients are understandable, appropriate, and might be important to answer (see chapter 7).

From our perspective, we feel that the less clients know about your private life, the better. In friendships, not disclosing personal information appears cold or impersonal; but in psychotherapy, too much therapist self-disclosure introduces impurities into the relationship. Thus, the virtues of honesty and openness need to be balanced with others, such as prudence and benevolence. For example, it may not be wise to share with your client your current relationship struggles or financial hardships. They can quickly interpret this type of sharing of information as an avenue to friendship with you which then leads to compromising the primary focus of the session – their goals and wellbeing.

Another example: if the client asks you about children and being in a marriage or significant relationship, they may be appropriately trying to get a handle on your "practical" experience of their issues. It might be appropriate and helpful to respond, "Yes, I have two children," or "Yes, I am married," and leave it at that. But even here, you need to be careful to bolster the boundary by not answering with too much personal information. You may also want to remind clients of your professional training and experience. If clients persist and ask you to tell them more about yourself, you may begin to suspect that your self-disclosure is satisfying other, nontherapeutic, needs of clients. Once again, your self-disclosure runs the risk of diminishing the true focus of therapy.

Clearly in most intimate personal relationships a high value is placed on transparency, honesty, and disclosure. However, as you move toward integration ask yourself these questions: Does your expertise and effectiveness come *primarily* from your personal life or from your professional training and experience? Does sharing information about your personal life lead to the best treatment outcomes (Foundation #1) and the most ethical behavior?

Your desire to self-disclose may be a very good indicator of some of your motivations. For example, if you feel you want to disclose more about yourself to a particular client than to others, you can take that as a red flag, and perhaps a violation of Ethical Foundation #4. Your desire to self-disclose may be the first evidence you have of your attraction to the client. We'd encourage you to stop and explore your motivations before you do any self-disclosure.

Here are three examples of how therapists might address questions about a personal issue, such as being a parent, partly based on their theoretical orientation: One therapist, coming from a psychoanalytic tradition (culture), might delay a direct answer and explore instead why the client is interested in how many children he has. He might say, "I'm wondering what makes you interested in that question." This comment or redirection is perfectly reasonable because psychotherapy is all about exploring motives and the focus should stay on the client. For some therapists, this response may be too much of an assimilation strategy in that it doesn't allow what they would consider a respectful answering of the question. For others, it would be much more comfortable.

Another therapist might take a more existential or humanistic approach and respond, "I have two children. I'm wondering if my answer changes anything." Some therapists might consider this response more respectful, and notice that the focus is quickly brought back to the client.

A third psychotherapist may respond somewhat unethically to the children question: "Oh! Let me show you pictures! Ronda's seven and Howard is two. Oh, they are so wonderful! Why, just yesterday ..." and then spend several minutes bragging to the client about the soccer games, and the chess club, and the trials and tribulations of potty training. In this interaction, the therapist is choosing an extreme separation strategy.

Your acculturation task is to find an appropriate response of honoring clients' desires to understand your personal experience while avoiding too much self-disclosure. As with all boundary issues, you need to consider variables such as the nature of the specific relationship, the client's gender, culture, age, and therapeutic goals, as well as your own values and tendencies.

Food for Thought: *Personal and Professional Considerations in Self-disclosure*

Think of a problem in your own life that you have recently dealt with. Now, imagine yourself in a therapy session and your client brings up the same problem that you have recently experienced. How tempted are you to disclose all or parts of your own story? Here are some questions to check your motivation:

- If I share my story (all or part), am I giving an example to show support or am I enjoying hearing myself talk?
- Can the focus of the session stay on the client or will it shift to me?
- Does the point of my story relate to the client's concerns?
- To what extent is the example helpful? To what extent would I just be rambling or bragging?

Now, rethink the situation. How might your thinking, feeling, and behavior change if:

- the client was of a different gender or sexual orientation;
- the client's problem was about a religious issue;
- you were very attracted, physically, to the client;

- the client was of a different cultural group;
- you were being observed by a student therapist;
- you were being observed by a supervisor.

Food for Thought: *Self-disclosure*

How self-disclosing are you as a person? How detailed do you get when you tell stories? How much information do you share about yourself in your close relationships and in your more formal relationships? It could be that you are very forthcoming and you bristle at the idea of not being able to "let it all hang out" with clients. Even the notion that some disclosures may be less therapeutic than others is new to you! It could be that you are very reserved, and you've thought about therapy as a professional relationship that hinges on technique and not personality. Now, you are faced with the clinical or ethical requirement that you disclose at least some information.

How do you think your "background level" of self-disclosure fits with the styles of the therapists described above? How might your preferences for self-disclosure fit within the different styles of psychotherapy that you know about? (For veteran therapists: How have your decisions about self-disclosure changed over the years? Why might that be?)

Touching: Crossing a Physical and Psychological Boundary

For sure, sexual touching between a therapist and client is never ethical, but other types of touch are up for debate. Some therapists take a very conservative view. They don't go beyond a handshake. These therapists do this, in part, because they see it as a way to show respect by treating clients equally (Foundation #4) and they believe it is impossible to know how clients will react to behaviors like a hug or an arm around the shoulder. This perspective might also be related to their culture of origin. Some people grow up in families where physical touch is rare. Alternatively, some therapists may greet clients with a hug, or sometimes give a client a literal pat on the back. Therapists who choose this behavior see it as a way to show warmth and caring. This too might be a reflection of their family of origin where everyone gets hugs as they come and go.

Food for Thought: *To Touch or Not to Touch*

Of course, therapists can never know for sure how a particular client is receiving their touch. But you can assess your own intent. Write down 4–5 situations in which you might consider touching a client in a variety of ways. Be specific about the situation, the characteristics of the client, and the type of touch.

To explore your own motivations and decisions for whom and how you touch, consider these questions for each scenario you wrote:

- Why do I touch? What am I trying to communicate through my touch?
- Whom do I touch?
- Is it only one gender? Or both?
- Do I touch only those who are physically appealing to me?
- How do I touch?
- Have I asked the client if my touch is comfortable or uncomfortable?

Now, rethink the situation. How might your thinking, feeling, and behavior change if:

- the client was of a different gender or sexual orientation;
- the client's problem was about a religious issue;

- you were very attracted, physically, to the client;
- the client was of a different cultural group;
- you were being observed by a student therapist;
- you were being observed by a supervisor.

Journal Entry: *Touch Continuum*

Draw a line across the middle of a piece of paper. On one end of the line put the words "Definitely Do Touch or Would Touch" and on the other end of the continuum put the words "Definitely Do Not Touch or Wouldn't Touch." At the midpoint of the line put a mark that shows the border between touching and not touching.

1. Now place the types of clients that fit along this continuum. For example, you may list opposite gender halfway along the "Wouldn't Touch" side, or "Child" all the way at the "Would Touch" end.
2. Share your continuum with someone else who is a colleague or fellow student. Discuss the reasons for your placement of types of clients.
3. Under what conditions might a particular client move from one side of the continuum to the other?
4. What type of touching did you have in mind when you considered the above questions? You might want to redo the questions while considering different types of touching.

Precursors to Boundary Violations

Some behaviors are *never* part of *any* therapeutic role and therapists are violating professional boundaries by engaging in such behavior. Here are some examples:

- engaging in sexual behavior with a client;
- financially exploiting a client;
- inviting a client to join you at your place of worship or a spiritual retreat;
- asking for more information about situations than is necessary.

All these boundary violations are disrespectful to clients (Foundation #3). They negate the trust you and your clients are trying to build. They will likely cause harm (Foundation #2), make clients feel emotionally and psychologically confused, and take the focus off of clients' goals. Here are a couple red flag stories that highlight these behaviors.

Red Flag: *Counterproductive Curiosity About Clients*

> When they were going over a traumatic event from her childhood, Ella understood that it was helpful to tell her story fully to her therapist, Dr Hunter. Now, however, no matter what topic Ella is discussing, Dr Hunter sits forward in her chair and asks for explicit details. Ella thinks, "Why is my therapist so interested in names, dates, locations, and sexual positions!"

Put yourself in the role of Dr Hunter and think about some of the motivations for doing therapy that you explored in chapter 1. As you review each of those motivations, think about where you would draw the line to stop asking questions. Focus in on the gray areas – what information would be both therapeutic to know as well as satisfy your motivation to learn interesting stories about people? Often the situations that fulfill both professional and personal motivations are the trickiest!

Red Flags: *Spiritual Selling, Invidious Invitations, and Shared Secrets Seem Suspicious*

Dr Pinkus has been seeing Ms Lateef for stress management for several weeks. At the end of one session, she wishes Dr Pinkus a happy Easter. "Where are you worshipping Easter?" asks Dr Pinkus.

"Oh, my husband and I don't belong to a church," replies Ms Lateef. As she says this she sees what can only be described as a dark cloud drift over Dr Pinkus's face.

"What a shame!" exclaims Dr Pinkus. "We would love to have you come to our church!"

Ms Lateef is taken aback. She has never raised the subject of religion during the therapy, and was only wishing Dr Pinkus a happy Easter just to be polite. This invitation seems too quick, too removed from therapy, and a little creepy. After all, Ms Lateef thinks, who is this "we" that she's talking about? Does she invite all her clients to her church? Does she tell her family or friends at her church that she invites clients to worship with them? "No, thanks," she manages to say.

Dr Pinkus says, "I think it's important to have a church to go to. If you came to mine we wouldn't have to tell anybody I'm your therapist. In fact, if anybody asks, it would be better if we just say that we're friends. Or, how about we pretend to be strangers and that you found the church in the phone book?"

Ms Lateef now feels herself getting angry. This isn't the kind of honesty that Dr Pinkus has been encouraging Ms Lateef to develop!

Perspectives on Multiple Relationships

Multiple relationships can be viewed as ongoing boundary crossings or violations that develop into identifiable relationships. Here is a short list of possible multiple relationships:

- being a therapist for a friend, relative, employee, and/or student;
- turning a client into a friend;
- taking on an evaluator role with a client (such as doing a custody evaluation for a client's child);
- entering into a business venture (other than the therapy, of course) with a client;
- entering into therapy with a person with whom you have had sexual relations.

Similar to self-disclosure and other boundary issues, there is a lively debate about the ethical nature of multiple relationships with clients – a continuum of perspectives. Of course, there are some multiple role relationships with clients that are universally seen as unethical, such as being in a dating or sexual relationship with a client. Other multiple role relationships (e.g., friendships with clients or being a dental patient of your client) are seen by some as appropriate, ethical, and just the way life is or should be (Lazarus & Zur, 2002).

On the end of the continuum where we happen to be, most multiple relationships are seen as problematic. Psychologist and ethics expert Karen Kitchener (2000) has written a lot about multiple relationships and their problematic nature. This is the way she explains it: In every relationship people play roles, and each role has a set of expectations (what others think we should do or be like) and a set of obligations (those things required of us). As ethical psychotherapists, we have role expectations and obligations with our clients. Consistent with our role expectations and obligations, we act in ways that ensure their wellbeing is our main concern (Foundation #1), we are obligated to keep their confidences (Foundation #3), we maintain boundaries (Foundation #7); in general, we plan to do our best work for clients.

If you and your clients enter into another type of relationship (for example, friends, business partners, or romantic partners), doing so introduces a whole new set of role expectations and obligations into the relationship. From our perspective, these new expectations and obligations compromise therapeutic relationships; therapists experience role strain and clients experience disequilibrium. For example, you may have a hard time honoring your professional obligations if you are also being a friend to your clients. In a friendship, both parties and their personal needs are of equal importance in the relationship, self-disclosure is engaged in by both parties, and both parties feel free to give and receive advice. Clients who are also your friends may very likely feel frustrated, confused, and angry trying to make sense of the role changes. At one point their needs are the priority but then the next time you are together, you and your needs are the focus.

Another problem with multiple relationships is that once you and the client get involved in the second relationship you can't really go back to just the therapy role. Think of the therapy relationship as a delicate flower in a greenhouse. If you take the delicate flower out of the greenhouse into a different environment, it will suffer or die. This is true of the therapy relationship; if you and your clients take it out of the therapy context, it will suffer and may die.

Like other boundary violations, multiple relationships can start as very simple behaviors or invitations that do not seem dramatic but that still compromise the purity and integrity of the therapy relationship. Beware of those subtle situations that appear benign but really violate the professional boundary (such as meeting for coffee) and that suggest another type of relationship. Although the invitation might seem small, innocent, and even courteous, it could be the beginning of a slippery slope to other types of interactions and a nontherapy, even exploitive, relationship.

We will be considering confidentiality in chapter 6, but we give you some coming attractions here in the context of boundaries and multiple relationships. As you read this story, you might want to make some notes in your journal about it – in addition to the ones we suggest below.

Green Flag: *Beneficial Boundary Bolstering,* *and* Red Flag: *Compromised Confidentiality*

Two psychotherapists walk into a bar. They find a quiet booth in the back and order imported light beers. "How's it going?" says Dr Greene.

"Not so good," says Dr Cherry. "I'm having trouble with a client."

Dr Greene says, "Before you tell me, remember to disguise the person's identity so you don't violate confidentiality."

"Sure," says Dr Cherry. "I won't tell you anything about him. Just that he lost his job in the computer industry, so I let him talk me into trading psychotherapy for his services as a web page designer."

"Don't you know that puts you in a multiple relationship?" said Dr Greene.

"Yeah, I thought about that. But it looked like a pretty straight-forward case. And how hard could it be to set up a web page for me? This guy said he'd done it before."

Dr Greene: "So what happened?"

Dr Cherry waits while the waiter sets the beers down and walks away, then says, "Well, pretty much anything that could go wrong has gone wrong. He turned out to have lots more to talk about in therapy than I thought, which means that even though he considers himself finished doing my web page, he still needs lots more therapy. If that were the only thing, it wouldn't be so bad, but the web page didn't even turn out like I wanted it to. He never really listened to what I wanted and just put up all these fancy bells and whistles. I just wanted a dignified 'CherryTreatment.com' site, but he has all these fancy colors and everything. And he won't even let me change it!"

Food for Thought: *Multiple Relationships*

Let's cut into the middle of this scenario for an exercise. As an ethical psychotherapist, Dr Cherry wants to be helpful to his client and he also has needs. But the unexpected happens – the contract doesn't work out. Dr Cherry's predicamen t can occur via behaviors that have the best of intentions. Let's go through and make an assessment of situation.

Part 1 Take the part of Dr Cherry and work through your choice-making process as you contemplate whether to enter into this contract and multiple role relationship with the client. Here are some questions to help.

- What are the good points of the decision?
- What are the bad points?
- What acculturation strategies might you be choosing?
- If you had the opportunity to do it over again, would you do anything differently? If no, why not? If yes, why so?

Part 2   Take the part of Dr Greene:

- What are you feeling and thinking as you're listening to Dr Cherry's description of his situation?
- From your perspective, what are the good points of the decision?
- What are the bad points?
- What might you encourage Dr Cherry to do now?

Part 3   Take the part of the client:

- What are you feeling and thinking about the contract?
- How are you feeling and thinking about your work on the web page?
- How are you feeling and thinking about your work in therapy?

Let's get back to the conclusion of our scenario. As you read through, continue to imagine yourself as each of the three characters and see if you can isolate the feelings, acculturation tasks, choice points, and options of all three:

> Dr Greene is angry and concerned. He's angry because his colleague should have known better, and these kinds of things reflect poorly on the entire profession. And he's concerned because neither Dr Cherry nor his client have benefited from this relationship. "This is exactly why you don't get into these multiple relationships. You can't predict what will go wrong, even when things appear simple and straightforward. It's just not worth the risk, either for you or for the client."
>
> Dr Cherry looks guilty. He responds, "But the client was so insistent!"

Dr Greene: "Look, who's the responsible party here? I know it seems like you were very respectful of the client's wishes. But clients aren't trained in ethics, and their wishes aren't always in their own best interests. It's part of your job to know the dangers, even if clients are insistent. I had one client who wanted to do repairs to my office one time. And I really needed those repairs done! But I just told him that the therapy would be much better if he just paid cash. And I told him what might go wrong, such as the work not being done the way I wanted it. He protested some, but he also understood when I made it clear that this was my general policy. It was nothing personal about him. That's one way to handle these situations."

Dr Cherry all of a sudden doesn't feel like finishing his beer. "You're right. I'm going to refer this client to another therapist."

Dr Greene is a bit relieved to see Dr Cherry taking some action to rectify the situation. A referral will be a little disruptive, but it'll probably give the client the best chance of getting some objective therapy.

They talk for a while about other things, and then leave the bar. When Dr Greene gets back to his office he gets on the web and looks up "CherryTreatment.com," just to see what it's like. Actually, the page doesn't look too bad. But when he gets down to the end, he is surprised and discouraged to see this in bright blue letters: "Web page designed by Moses Demm."

Even When Therapy Is Over, the Relationship Lives On

At this point you might be thinking, "OK, I see your point about multiple role relationships during therapy. But what about when therapy is over? We can be friends (or lovers, or business partners, or ...), right?"

We don't think so! Opinions vary on this, but we believe that, although therapy has ended, the therapeutic relationship still continues inside clients (and you) on a psychological level (Buckley, Karasu, & Charles, 1981; Anderson & Kitchener, 1996). To enter into another relationship would thus create a multiple role. Besides, if you have done some good work with the client, she or he may want to resume therapy in the future. If the temptation arises to initiate another relationship with your client, this is a perfect time to invoke the *Why Bother* rule. That is: Why bother doing something ethically questionable when you will only increase the likelihood of future problems? Why not act more positively and pursue ethical excellence? Good therapy is very difficult at best for both therapists and clients. It is a big investment on both sides. Why complicate things and disrupt what you have accomplished?

Food for Thought: *Posttermination Relationships*

Choose three nontherapy relationships that you might choose to have (or find yourself in inadvertently) with a former client. Rank-order them in terms of the risk of harm to the former client, and your confidence that pursuing such a relationship is a bad (or good) idea.

Now, vary the following characteristics of the therapeutic relationship and see if these factors, alone or in combination, change your judgments (these characteristics are based on Gottlieb, 1993):

- the duration of treatment (one hour, ten years, etc.);
- the definiteness of termination ("We've completed our ten-session systematic desensitization," "Come back any time," etc.);
- the power differential in therapy (long-term psychoanalysis, limited smoking-cessation treatment, etc.);
- the functioning of the client (perfect mental health, lingering transference, etc.);
- the cultural identification of the client;
- the attractiveness of the client (physically, emotionally, etc.)

One final question: As you weighed the factors that might influence your decision, how sure can you be that you can determine what might happen? For example, how sure can you be about the future plans of clients?

Of course there are times when posttherapy relationships are unavoidable. For example, you and your former client might find yourselves on the same committee at your child's school or part of the same social/professional network. When this happens, it is important to make good acculturation choices, recognizing your professional obligations, personal values and motivations, and the likelihood of harm (Anderson & Kitchener, 1998).

Flashing Yellow Sign: Slippery Slope Ahead

You know how – when you are driving along and in the distance you begin to see a flashing yellow light – your foot automatically comes off the accelerator pedal? That reaction happens because you become aware or you've been alerted to some situation ahead that is problematic. Just like that yellow flashing light, there are signs or signals to be aware of as a professional to keep from starting down the slippery slope. Here are some of them:

- Personal stress. Life happens to us, too. Get your own help via your own therapist.
- Professional or career stress. There are bills to pay and obligations to meet. Take time for self-care so that clients get your best. Also, finances or financial problems can prompt us to make unethical decisions (keeping clients in therapy when therapy is over, falsifying insurance forms to get payment, etc.).
- Life changes. We all go through different life stages and changes. With each one a new set of challenges and possible benefits come. For example, think about these life events:
  - death of a loved one;
  - marriage;
  - end of a significant relationship;
  - moving to another location, far from a usual support group;
  - serious illness;
  - sexual problems;
  - major change in financial status.

If these situations begin to overwhelm us and we do not seek the support we need, several things can happen. Here are just a few: we become impaired in our professional performance, our clients do not receive our best, *we* become very vulnerable to boundary violations, or we enter multiple role relationships that can do irreparable harm.

Inadvertent Contact

Contact outside of therapy will happen; is this always a problem? It does not have to be. For example, there are times when boundary crossings happen accidentally: You see your client at the grocery store or a concert, your child is on the same soccer team as your client's child, or you happen to be guests at the same party. These situations happen, especially – but not only – in small communities.

For these accidental contacts to occur is one thing. How you handle them is another. Of course, you would have the sense to not violate the therapeutic relationship by announcing at the party, "Hey, look who's here – my favorite client!" On the other hand, clients may be really confused if you choose to ignore them all evening and act as if they are not even there.

One way to prevent these crossings from being harmful (and even to provide some therapeutic benefit) is for you and your clients to discuss the possible crossings. In fact, when you anticipate that such crossings might occur (for example, in a small community), you can talk about it beforehand and decide how you want to handle the situation. One good approach is called the *You First* arrangement (Knapp & VandeCreek, 2006). Consider the party scenario. Using the "You First" strategy, you will leave it up to the client to initiate contact, say hello, introduce you to others, or whatever. But if the client does not initiate it, then no contact or no recognition occurs. This is a good arrangement because the issue has been discussed beforehand and clients maintain control over the situation.

Being a Therapist for Someone You Already Know

As we mentioned previously, working with someone you know might be a wonderful thing to do in other relationships. For example, when you are looking to have some major improvements done on your house, or you are considering a major purchase, you often want to work with someone whom you already have some trust in or knowledge about. This person might be a neighbor on the next street or someone you have met at the bridge club or on the tennis courts. As we have seen, however, being a therapist and having some prior knowledge or experience with a person can taint or skew the work that needs to be done. As the therapist you need to be clear-headed and objective about what or how to help the client. If you work with a friend, you might be tempted not to challenge them so much or confront them about their issues.

A gray area: Let's say you have an acquaintance who seeks your services as a psychotherapist. For example, you might live in the same small community, or be a member of a church or a member of the gay community and your clientele is from this network. Or you might be a psychology instructor or workshop presenter and one of your students or participants asks for your card because they want to make an appointment for therapy. An assimilation strategy might be to flatly reject the role of therapist: "I can't have any other relationship." A separation strategy might be to accept the invitation immediately: "Of course! We already have lots in common!" A more integrative and positive strategy would be to talk through the new relationship with the prospective client so that all the parties understand the expectations and obligations with the new roles. At this point you can make a better decision about how to respond. If you decide to be a therapist, you will have started by providing good information about the boundaries of this relationship (see chapter 7). If you decide to decline the request, you can still provide useful guidance (as any friend would) about how to find a more appropriate therapist.

Green Flag: *Responsible Referrals*

After you read this scenario, speculate about the acculturation influences and choices of Dr Ruiz:

> Norah is seeing Dr Ruiz and the therapy is going well. Dr Ruiz notices that Norah is talking about different kinds of life choices,

career issues, time management, and stuff that could really be done by coaching rather than therapy. Dr Ruiz considers switching from therapy to coaching, and offering Norah her coaching skills. After all, she's been trained to be a coach in addition to her therapy training. But then Dr Ruiz has two thoughts that save her and Norah from a boundary violation. First, Dr Ruiz thinks, "Wait; if I do coaching, it'll get in the way of our good therapy work." Second, Dr Ruiz thinks, "Why am I so arrogant to think that I am the only person who can provide coaching to Norah?"

At the end of the next session, Dr Ruiz says, "Norah, I notice that there are some issues you are talking about that might be well suited to explore with a life coach. Here is a list of three local people who do life coaching. You may want to think about that option."

Norah says, "But, Dr Ruiz, you are trained as a life coach, right?"

"Yes."

"So, why can't you coach me? You already know a lot about me," Norah asks, reasonably.

Just a faint touch of a smile crosses Dr Ruiz's face as she thinks to herself, "In graduate school they said I'd get questions like this from clients, and I didn't believe them!" Out loud, she says, "Norah, coaching is quite a different activity, and if we switched to do that, I can't guarantee that the therapy we've been working so hard at would be as good. It's a much better idea, I think, if we keep working like we have been, and you see somebody who can devote all their energies to coaching. Does that make sense? Think about working with a life coach; there's no need to make up your mind right now."

Journal Entry: *Acculturating to Boundaries*

As a way to recap your explorations in this chapter, we invite you to create a catalogue of boundary crossings and violations from this chapter and explore your acculturation strategies to each. Here is your task:

1. Make a list of all the examples of boundary crossings/violations in this chapter.
2. *Add* to that list a number of behaviors that you would consider crossings/violations. To help you generate these examples, think about your own hobbies, previous jobs, political and religious views, and personal relationships.
3. For each example, write two short vignettes, one of which is a harmless (or beneficial) boundary crossing and the other a harmful violation.
4. For each of these vignettes, add a list of your potential motivations, including personal and professional, appropriate and inappropriate.
5. For each vignette, consider several courses of action, including unethical choices, preventive measures, and ways to deal with a situation in which the crossing/violation has already occurred.
6. For each course of action, think about the acculturation strategy that seems predominant. See if you can "fix" some of the actions by using more integration strategies – by explicitly recognizing the elements of your decision that come from your own background and the culture of psychotherapy.

Conclusion

Some might say that we (Sharon and Mitch) are conservative and rigid on this issue of relationship boundaries in psychotherapy. We are definitely on the side of the continuum that encourages psychotherapists to avoid multiple relationships with clients. We acknowledge that it is a good sign when your client enjoys you as their therapist, appreciates your work, and wishes to have you more involved in their life. But we say, "Don't go there. You are already ahead of the game." Even if the client begs, pleads with, or pursues you for something more, it is still your responsibility to say, *"No, thank you! I want to just be your therapist."*

6

Confidentiality

A Critical Element of Trust
in the Relationship

Consider this story from Sharon:

> As a mom of two children who love movies, I have seen my fair
> share of Disney pictures – some of them multiple times. To be
> honest, I don't mind seeing *Aladdin* over again. I like the main plot
> (the orphaned peasant boy wins the hand of a beautiful young
> princess) and watch with interest the exploration of two other
> themes: the battle of good against evil and the struggle just to be
> oneself. Another theme in *Aladdin*, and one that Mitch and I kept
> returning to as we designed this chapter, is trust. In two different
> scenes, Aladdin extends his hand to Jasmine and asks, "Do you
> trust me?" meaning, "Are you willing to take a risk with me?" In
> the first scene the risk is to jump off a building to escape from the
> palace guards who are in hot pursuit. In the second, it's to take a
> ride on Aladdin's magic carpet. In both scenes, Jasmine reaches
> out to grab hold of his hand, indicating that she does trust him.

Therapy is no magic carpet, but it certainly involves clients taking
risks and being able to trust the therapist. At the core of a therapist's
offer of trust (the figuratively extended hand of the therapist) is the
issue of confidentiality. Without the promise and commitment of confidentiality, the trustworthiness of the therapist is not a viable possibility.
As therapists, we are there to hear all that the client might wish to share
and to both implicitly and explicitly promise, "I will keep your information confidential."

Confidentiality can be defined most simply as "the obligation of
professionals to respect the privacy of clients and the information they
provide" (Handelsman, 1987, p. 33). Confidentiality is based on the

constitutional right of privacy – you and I have the right to decide who knows what about us when (Kitchener, 2000). This obligation is such a critical element in the psychotherapy relationship that some authors have referred to confidentiality as a "sacred covenant" (Driscoll, 1992, p. 704), a bedrock promise. Keeping the confidences of clients is one of the major role obligations of psychotherapists and a hallmark of the culture of psychotherapy. Although the obligation to maintain confidentiality is supported by several of our Ethical Foundations, it is important enough to have one of its own (Foundation #8).

Clients may feel a push–pull about our promise of confidentiality. On the one hand, they want to accept the offer of confidentiality – to trust the therapist – and to be able to share all that they think and feel inside without any hesitation. On the other hand, they may be unfamiliar with such promises and fear the possibility that the therapist will (a) judge the personal information that they hear, or (b) disclose the clients' confidences to colleagues, spouses, or others. Could a total stranger really keep their private feelings and thoughts safe?

You might be thinking, "OK, I thought the *Aladdin* movie was entertaining and, yes, confidentiality is a major way to demonstrate trustworthiness. But what's with all the drama? I keep the secrets of my friends all the time. No big deal!" As we will explore in this chapter, your acculturation task regarding confidentiality may just be a bit more stressful than you think. To have clients be able to say anything at all – no matter how embarrassing or deeply personal – and have the statements valued, respected, and protected from disclosure is one of the things that differentiate the culture of therapy from other types of relationships. There are certainly some similarities between confidentiality in therapy and privacy in friendships; for example, the giver of information is hoping for his or her information to stay private and the relationship would be damaged if the promise is not upheld. However, as we explore the complexities of confidentiality and the critical nature of trust in the professional relationship, the differences should become crystal clear.

Let's turn up the acculturation temperature a little bit: As we present confidentiality as a cornerstone of the therapeutic relationship, we hasten to add that the promise of confidentiality in therapy is not absolute. Partly for this reason, dilemmas and issues revolving around confidentiality are among the most common dilemmas therapists face (Pope & Vetter, 1992).

In this chapter we will help you develop your sensitivity to the true essence of client confidentiality. Our experience in working with students – and some professionals already in the field – tells us that "culture-of-origin" ideas about privacy are usually *not* enough to consistently honor the principle of confidentiality in psychotherapy. For example, a couple of years ago during a class discussion on confidentiality, Sharon remembers a student being very honest and saying, "This keeping secrets and confidentiality thing will really be tough. I am naturally nosy and I like to share good stories."

In addition to helping you develop your sensitivity to confidentiality, we will also help you acknowledge and increase your tolerance for uncomfortable feelings when confidentiality has to be breached. Breaking the client's confidentiality when it's necessary is probably one of the more heart-wrenching and uncomfortable tasks a psychotherapist has to face. This is especially true for new professionals and students in practicum or internship settings.

Sensitivity and Understanding of Confidentiality

Personal – Your Preexisting Culture about Confidentiality

To begin this section, let's explore your ethics of origin. More specifically, let's look at aspects of your preexisting "confidentiality culture" with an eye toward deciding which aspects will be worth maintaining and which may be incompatible with the culture of psychotherapy.

Journal Entry: *Me and Secrets*

We would like you to write about four actual or potential situations from your life.

First situation Consider a time when you told someone something very personal and you expected them to keep this information to themselves. However, they didn't keep your secret and told someone else your personal information. If you cannot think of a particular instance, speculate about an incident that *could* have happened in your life. Answer these questions:

- How does it feel to have your personal information shared?
- What happened (or might have happened) to the relationship between the two of you?

Second situation   Consider a time when you shared personal information with someone else and (at least to your knowledge) they kept your secret.

- What does that feel like?
- What was (is) the relationship like with that person?
- What was (is) it about that person, do you think, that helps them honor your confidences?
- Write about some of the similarities and differences between your first two situations. You might write about the context, the relationships, your feelings, or the other person's motives for sharing or keeping your secret.

Third situation   Let's turn the tables and have you reflect about yourself in the "secret keeper" role. Write about a time when you've kept a secret that was told to you by somebody, even when you experienced some temptation to share it. Write the story and then answer these questions:

- What were your feelings?
- What was the temptation like and what did it feel like to keep the confidence?
- What did you tell yourself that enabled you to keep the secret? That is, how did you justify your decisions?
- What is the relationship like now?

Fourth situation   Write about a time when someone shared something personal with you and they expected you to keep their confidence but you ended up sharing the information with a third party.

- What happened?
- Why did you share the information?

- What did it feel like to make the decision and carry it out? (If you feel like you shared the information without a conscious decision, we encourage you to think again!)
- What happened to the relationship between you and that person?
- Why were you not able to keep this secret while being able to keep the other one?

Having considered and written about these four examples, here are some other general questions to consider:

- Look back at the values journal entry ("Values, Nothing More than Values") that you completed in chapter 1. Did anything like privacy, confidentiality, or respecting others' information show up on your list? If not, where would you put respect for privacy now?
- Are you a natural story teller? (If you're not sure, ask your friends. If you're still not sure, ask your enemies!)
- If you are a natural story teller, what benefits do you get out of this role? What drawbacks does it have?

We make decisions every day about what personal information of ours we want to share with others, and the kinds of information that others have shared with us that we pass along. Many of the decisions we make are second nature; we may not even realize that we have rules about what to share with whom, when. As an exercise, identify a specific person in each of the categories of people we've listed below. If you can't – you don't have an attorney, for example – think about another person who plays a similar role in your life (e.g., your accountant):

- a parent
- a distant cousin
- an acquaintance
- your closest friend
- your spouse/partner/significant other
- your attorney
- your physician
- your clergyperson

Now, think about some types of personal information you would or would not share with each of these people. For example, to whom among the above individuals and under what conditions might you tell them:

- a store you shop at that you are a little embarrassed about?
- an incident in childhood that you'd rather forget?
- a sexual behavior or position you've always wanted to try but haven't?
- your hopes and dreams for the future?

Now, consider each of these people telling *you* these things. What would your reaction be?

Professional – Confidentiality in the Psychotherapy Culture

It should be apparent by now that issues of privacy and confidentiality are complex in our normal negotiation of relationships. When we look toward acculturating to the psychotherapy culture, the picture might appear a bit clearer, but only for a while. Read on …

We start with several characteristics of confidentiality in psychotherapy that are critical to understand, especially in a positive approach. One key aspect of confidentiality is that *everything* said between a client and a therapist is confidential, no matter how dull or routine it might be (Welfel, 2006), and no matter how good it might be as a story for your next get-together with friends. What we might think is mundane and ordinary and unnecessary to keep as a confidence, clients might see as very private, personal parts of themselves. As Welfel (2006) suggests,

> Zealously guarding client privacy also indicates a true compassion for the courage it takes for clients to enter treatment. … Honoring confidentiality requires integrity precisely because it can be difficult – the human tendency to want to share experiences does not bypass mental health professionals simply because they have a credential. (p. 67)

We have heard something like this from more than one student, "Wow, I tell my partner everything. You mean, now I have to keep secrets from them?" Our response is, "Yes, absolutely!" You need to set and keep a boundary with significant others in your life about client confidentiality. Your spouse, partner, and best friends are not meant to be the beneficiaries of interesting stories from clients. Nor are they entitled to be privy to that level of detail about your work.

Psychotherapists who choose a separation strategy might argue, "Come on. My client tells me about their favorite restaurant and this is considered confidential? It won't do any harm to share that information with my spouse!" Although it seems picky and extreme not to be able to share such a trivial tidbit, a promise of confidentiality is a promise of confidentiality. It is true that the risk of harm is quite low in this example, but the underlying principle goes beyond doing good (Foundation #1) and avoiding harm (Foundation #2) to Foundation #3: "Treat clients with respect." Bok (1989) encourages us to remember that keeping our promise with the small and trivial issues shows the client that we can be trusted with the more important matters they disclose. It also expresses our virtues (Foundation #10) of diligence, prudence, and integrity. Although there are exceptions to confidentiality which we discuss shortly, it might be good to think of the default option as keeping everything a client says confidential unless there is a clear reason to disclose the information, rather than seeing every disclosure of a client as possible material for our next friendly conversation over dinner.

A second difference between confidentiality in psychotherapy and other relationships is the assumption made by clients (Welfel, 2006). Typically, clients assume that what they share is confidential. As a result they don't bother to stop and say, "You'll keep this just between the two of us, right?" which is what a friend would likely do with another friend. If clients need always to be thinking about how we might use their information outside of therapy, they are taking precious time and energy away from the work of therapy. Like boundary crossings, this is a contaminating factor in the fragile psychotherapeutic relationship.

A third difference is that confidentiality in therapy extends all the way to revealing a client's identity (Welfel, 2006). As we mentioned in chapter 3, keeping the client's identity private is referred to as *contact confidentiality* (Ahia & Martin, 1993). As psychotherapists we have the obligation to keep our clients' identities unknown to others. The following is an example of (among other problems) not honoring a client's identity.

Red Flag: *Compromised Confidentiality*

> Dr Bechet is dedicated to helping her clients. … One day she says to one of her clients, Mr Armstrong, "Listen, I think you and Marion, one of my other clients, would get along splendidly! Here's her phone number."
>
> "Wha'?" says Mr. Armstrong. "I don't think this is –"
>
> "Oh, don't worry. Marion is always looking to meet men, and she has such trouble. And I think you'd be great for each other."
>
> Mr Armstrong is taken aback. Even though, he admits to himself, he's a little curious about this woman, he wonders how he's ever going to learn how to meet people if his therapist insists on playing matchmaker. And did Marion give her permission to have her number given to him? "No, thanks," he says, "I'd prefer not to." Mr Armstrong makes no move to accept the small piece of paper with the neatly written name and number on it.
>
> "Come on, take the number. Besides," continues Dr Bechet, "I've already given your number to her …"

Definitely Dr Bechet is not keeping or maintaining confidentiality! We might not cross the boundary as blatantly as Dr Bechet, but even the small things like sharing our day with our significant other or talking to clients in the hallway or waiting area indicates that we don't really understand the true essence or promise of confidentiality. How, or under what conditions, might you be most likely to infringe on clients' confidentiality?

Journal Entry: *Compromised Confidentiality*

As you read this next story, put yourself in the position of the narrator and the psychologist, and try to imagine – in writing – how both parties felt and what their options are:

My daughter and I are seeing a child/family psychotherapist. I think he's good with my child. But … It's like our fourth or fifth visit, and he's in a practice with other people, so they have this common waiting room. And my daughter and I get there and we're sittin' in the lobby area. And there's three other people. He comes out, you know, and says, "Is there anything I need to know about?" 'Cause he's gonna work with my daughter. So I just kind of give him some general stuff, you know, in front of these three other people I don't know!

So he takes my daughter back and he works with her. And then all of a sudden it hits me: Wow, that didn't feel too good! And then I laughed, like, I should know these things, I'm a mental health professional myself! But now I'm on the client side.

When I got home, I called him and left a message on his machine and said, "It didn't feel real good when you asked the question, 'Is there anything I need to know?' out in the lobby. That does not feel comfortable to me. I want to be able to go back in your office and address whatever I need to."

He called back the next morning and we kind of talked about the lobby thing. His first thing was, "Well, I hope you didn't see that as unprofessional behavior." In my head, I'm thinking, "Yeah! I did!" Because it was!

He said, "I didn't mean for you to disclose anything you wouldn't want to." I said, "Well, from now on I just want to go back into your office and have our conversation in there."

It's interesting, even as a psychotherapist it took me a little while to articulate what my discomfort was.

Food for Thought: *Why Do We Feel the Need to Share Client Information?*

Make a list of your possible motivations for disclosing information. Put yourself in positions where you *could* disclose information, then think about why you *would*. What reactions would you get? What feelings would you have? Whom would you please?

Can We Ever Say Anything?

When we promise confidentiality and then fail to keep it (when it should be kept), we are showing a lack of respect, integrity, and trustworthiness. But are there limits to our promise? Is there anything we can say to others about what we do in psychotherapy without violating our promise? As we discussed in chapter 3, people will ask you, "How'd it go today?" We cannot violate our promise of confidentiality. Neither, however, can we totally sacrifice our own personalities, mental health, and relationships. In other words, we need to work out some assimilation and integration strategies.

One common way to handle this situation is to talk about our feelings as a therapist without sharing identities of or personal information about our clients. We can talk to our significant others about how splendidly our day went and share the joys and frustrations of being a therapist. We can talk to colleagues about various types of clients who frustrate us. If we need consultation on a particular case, however, we would need to get the permission of our clients to get that consultation.

Sometimes both the therapist and client agree that information from therapy should be shared with others, including physicians and other professionals, work supervisors, clients' family members, and others. In these cases, we get our client's written permission to share information with appropriate professionals. The client has the power to give us permission to talk with others. That is, they waive their right to confidentiality through signing a *Release of Information* form that specifies who is involved and for how long we have that permission.

Green Flag: *Requests for Written Releases*

As you read this story, think about the virtues Dr Tall is displaying:

"Have you been in therapy before?" Dr Tall asks Jane.

"Oh, yes; I saw a psychiatrist last year for medication. But I didn't like the side effects."

"I think it would be a good idea if I talked to your previous psychiatrist. I would also like to talk with your physician, given the physical complaints you have."

"Sure! Talk with any of those folks. I'll give you their names and numbers."

"That's great; I'll just need you to sign a couple of release forms. It'll only take a few minutes."

Jane fidgets a bit in her chair. "Oh, we don't need forms. I already gave you my permission, and I trust you."

Dr Tall is not fazed. "It's not really a matter of trust. The forms help to refresh our memories and also give you the opportunity to change your mind."

"So, what exactly am I signing?"

"This form says that I can share information with your psychiatrist for purposes of your treatment. That means I won't just gossip! And the expiration date is six months from today, so if I need to talk with him after that, I'll ask you to renew your permission."

"And you said I could change my mind?"

"Sure. For any reason. It usually doesn't happen, but you have that right. Just tell me you don't want me to talk to him any more, and I'll make a note in your chart. And, by the way, we'll fill one of these out for each person, and I'll give you a copy of each of the forms, so you know what permissions you gave."

There are other situations in which sharing some information may be acceptable. For example, when we teach, we often use examples of cases we see for instructional purposes. The professions recognize the importance of teaching and the importance of using examples that capture the reality of therapy. We are allowed, therefore, to use our clinical case material as an illustration. However, when we teach we must disguise the identities of our clients (or, of course, get their permission, which is often clinically contraindicated).

Food for Thought: *To Breach or Not to Breach*

Once upon a time there was a psychotherapist, Dr D. Lemmah, who had been seeing a female client, Elaine, for several months. They had been making good progress and Elaine was gaining some wonderful insights into her history of failed relationships with men. One day Elaine comes into the session with a little smile on her face. She sits down and immediately starts to talk to Dr Lemmah about this new young man she met the other day, Jerry. She's already been out on a couple dates with Jerry, she says, and things are going quite well. She really thinks she's made some improvement in her relating to men! As she talks in more detail about her dates with Jerry, Dr Lemmah notices a slight ringing in his ears along with an uneasy feeling that starts in his head and travels down to the abdomen, and finally settles as a definite sinking feeling in the stomach. Jerry had been a client of Dr Lemmah's, having terminated two years ago. Jerry had made some progress with his depression and anxiety, but Dr Lemmah remembers that Jerry had been charged with a felony – physically abusing his (Jerry's) ex-wife.

Here are some questions to help you explore your reactions to this case. Be as explicit as you can in your responses:

1. What are your feelings toward or about Dr Lemmah, Elaine, and Jerry? Whom do you sympathize with the most? With whom do you identify the most?
2. If you were a friend of Elaine's and she told you her story about Jerry (and you knew what Dr Lemmah knew about him), what would you tell her?

Put yourself in Dr Lemmah's place:

3. What are your obligations to Elaine? To Jerry? To your profession?
4. What are your options for how to proceed?

5. Suppose you knew nothing about Jerry: How would you proceed in therapy with Elaine?

6. If you breach Jerry's confidentiality by telling Elaine about him and suggest she not see him, what is the likelihood that you will be successful in keeping them apart?

7. What do you decide to do? Why?

8. What facts of the case would have to be different for you to choose other options?

Put yourself in Jerry's place:

9. What would you expect Dr Lemmah to do in this case? Why?

10. How do you feel about Dr Lemmah's decision?

Put yourself in Elaine's place:

11. What would you expect Dr Lemmah to do in this case? Why?

12. How might you feel about Dr Lemmah's decision?

13. What have you learned – what therapeutic progress have you made – by what Dr Lemmah decided to do?

14. What would you like Dr Lemmah to tell his future clients about *you*?

Put yourself in the place of an ethics committee member:

15. The committee receives a complaint about Dr Lemmah from Elaine, who recently broke up with Jerry. During their breakup, it became apparent that Jerry was a former client of Dr Lemmah, and Elaine was furious that Dr Lemmah did not tell her about him weeks before. She believes Dr Lemmah acted unethically by not informing her of his knowledge about Jerry and insisting that she break up with Jerry immediately. What does the committee decide and on what grounds?

16. The committee receives a complaint about Dr Lemmah from Jerry, with whom Elaine recently broke up. During their breakup, it became apparent that Elaine was a client of Dr Lemmah and that he strongly suggested that Elaine end her relationship with Jerry. Jerry is furious. He believes Dr Lemmah acted unethically by breaching his confidentiality and incompetently by telling Elaine what to do rather than simply exploring her decisions. What does the committee decide and on what grounds?

Work through all these questions (1–16) again under the following conditions:

- Jerry is of an ethnic group you know very little about. If truth be known, you harbor some uncomfortable feelings toward this group.
- Elaine is really Edward and Jerry is Jayne. How does the change in genders change your gut reactions and professional judgments?

Final questions:

- What conflicts (of motives, values, virtues, and principles) were the most salient for you?
- What did you notice about your integrating your ethics of origin and your professional responsibilities? For example, did you reorganize your values to allow one to become more prominent? Did you shift your ideas about how to implement your values?

Breaching Confidentiality

As we mentioned before, confidentiality is not absolute. There are times when confidentiality cannot and should not be kept. The promise to respect clients' confidences comes with exceptions that need to be stated to the client in clear terms at the start of the therapy relationship. (We'll cover more about this in chapter 7.) These exceptions revolve around the safety of clients and/or others.

To understand the rationale behind the exceptions we can look at the major ethical rationale for confidentiality: the principle of autonomy (Foundation #3; Kitchener, 2000). Respecting client autonomy means (among other things) that clients have the right to choose who will know what about them when. However, the right to such autonomy is limited when that right infringes on the rights of others. For example, if a client indicates in therapy that he is planning on killing another individual, the psychotherapist has the ethical – and, in most states, the legal – responsibility to warn the potential victim of the possible harm as well as contact the police and possibly even get the client hospitalized for a psychiatric evaluation (Tarasoff, 1976). Likewise, if a client threatens to kill himself or herself, you are obligated to break confidentiality to save the client's life.

Breaching confidentiality to prevent a murder or a suicide is a clear instance of overriding a client's privacy for the purpose of preventing a terrible harm. But how serious does the harm have to be before we are justified in breaking confidentiality? Before we talk about the limits to confidentiality in more detail, we would like to give you an opportunity to explore potential difficult situations where you think confidentiality might need to be breached.

Journal Entry: *Once More into the Breach*

Consider each of the following situations and answer the following questions for each one: (a) What is your gut feeling about what you would *like* to do in each case? (b) Does your course of action involve a breach of confidentiality? (c) What courses of action are possible? (d) What does the profession (according to your other texts, professor, colleagues, ethics code) think about whether you should violate confidentiality? (e) What would you choose to do and why?

In therapy, a client tells you that he or she:

1. is feeling sad and sometimes wishes he or she were dead;
2. is really angry with a former partner;
3. is having an affair;
4. has robbed a store;
5. plans to embezzle money from the bank for which he or she works;
6. plans to embezzle money from the bank for which he or she works, which happens to be *your* bank;
7. drinks and is underage;
8. is engaged in touching children sexually;
9. had engaged in touching children sexually 30 years ago, but doesn't any more;
10. has tested positive for HIV and is having unprotected sex.

Now look at your answers. Which situations prompted the most discomfort? What virtues, principles, ethics codes and other sources of guidance did you call upon to make your professional decisions? What dimensions stand out, as you look at the pattern of your responses, in your decision-making? Was it only that some harm was done? The type of harm (e.g., physical vs. financial)? The amount of harm? The imminence of the harm? What happened when children were involved?

Limits to Confidentiality

Confidentiality is both an ethical and legal concept. All the professional codes address the issue of confidentiality and many states have laws that identify the term *legal confidentiality*, which mandates that conversations between a client and psychotherapist cannot be shared with another individual without legal ramifications (Cottone & Tarvydas, 2007).

The limits on, or exceptions to, confidentiality are prescribed by state statute, case law, and administrative law. The homicidal threats we talked about before are grounds for violating confidentiality in most states, as is the situation of suicide. All states have laws about reporting child abuse, although they vary regarding some of the parameters of such reporting. For example, in some states the situation in #9 in the previous journal entry would have to be reported – in other states, not. Some states require reporting of elder abuse, others do not. States vary also about whether minors are guaranteed confidentiality.

In addition to laws, agencies have their own policies about confidentiality. In an important sense, each agency represents a miniculture, with its own codes, traditions, and values.

Food for Thought: *Spouse Abuse*

Do you think spouse abuse should be a reportable offense? That is, if you find out that one spouse is physically abusive, should you report that to the authorities? Justify your answer in terms of virtues, values, principles, etc. Then, justify an *opposing* point of view.

The acculturation tasks regarding the limits of confidentiality may be quite stressful. How are we to move toward integration? Some of you may feel that these exceptions are too much – therapy should be treated as sacred; psychotherapists cannot take on police functions (Siegel, 1979). Indeed, coming to therapy where you are guaranteed a place to work out your problems in total privacy may actually reduce the total number of crimes committed in the population (this argument was the minority opinion in the Tarasoff [1976] decision). Those of you with these types of beliefs might adopt a separation strategy and be rather slow to break confidentiality even when such a violation is obligatory, as in the case of child abuse.

Another possible response to learning of these exceptions to confidentiality is that the exceptions do not go far enough! You might be among those whose ordinary moral sense would suggest calling the police to report a robbery or embezzlement by your clients, which are actions that do *not* need to be reported.

It may be difficult to violate confidentiality even when it is clearly justified. Indeed, many therapists report difficulty – acculturation stress, if you will – when dealing with these issues (Pope & Vetter, 1992). As psychotherapists, we have "offered our hand" to our client saying that we will be trustworthy and keep their secrets. When the situation or conversation suggests that we must violate confidentiality – even when we've told our clients the limits of our promise – our minds and hearts feel the conflict acutely. How do we choose integration strategies that allow us to preserve and violate confidentiality when necessary? One general strategy is to keep three thoughts in mind. First, the welfare of the client (or the intended victim of a serious threat, or the child in the case of child abuse) may be the highest principle. Second, we may not be the final arbiters – or providers – of that welfare. Third, the way we implement our ethical obligation, whether it is to violate or preserve confidentiality, is critical.

Another important part of your decision-making should be consultation. Consultation, peer supervision, and other ways to share and get feedback on your professional decisions can really help. Indeed, in many states you can be charged with unprofessional conduct if you fail to get consultation.

It's a Small World After All

Sometimes confidentiality is compromised through no fault of our own. Our world is smaller than we think; there may be times when we accidently end up seeing our client in another context like a grocery store or a concert. Our child may wind up on the same soccer team as our client's child, or we happen to be guests at the same party. These situations happen, especially (but not only) in small communities. How we handle these situations is important and communicates to the client our respect for the professional relationship. It is important to discuss these possible events occurring and decide how to handle them, such as the "You First" arrangement (Knapp & VandeCreek, 2006) that we mentioned in chapter 5.

Privilege and Confidentiality

Sometimes the terms *privilege* and *confidentiality* are seen as the same and used interchangeably in conversation by psychotherapists (Welfel, 2006). In actuality, they are two very different terms and come from two very, very different cultures. As we have discussed, confidentiality is both an ethical and legal obligation of the psychotherapist to maintain the conversation between the client and therapist and the identity of the client in confidence. *Privilege* and *privileged communication* are exclusively legal terms. Privilege is the right of the (adult) client to keep any communication that occurs in therapy from being revealed in legal proceedings (Cottone & Tarvydas, 2007). All 50 states include some form of client–psychotherapist privilege (Welfel, 2006). Once again, however, state law varies and some psychotherapeutic relationships may not be covered in all states.

Similar to confidentiality, the right of privileged communication has limitations. In a civil proceeding, the judge can issue a court order to have the therapist share information or produce client records. At this point, of course, prudent therapists get legal consultation to help them navigate this new culture. Appeals to the ruling can be filed, requesting that a higher court hear the psychotherapist's assertion of privileged communication, or the psychotherapist can decide to deal with the legal ramifications of refusing to cooperate with the court order.

Red Flag: *Porous Privacy*

Porous privacy occurs when therapists share information about one client with another individual or individuals without consent. This itself is a violation of confidentiality (Foundation #8), and it can be seen as disrespectful (Foundation #3) and potentially harmful (Foundation #2). The most problematic version of this behavior is a full disclosure, with names and/or other identifying information about some experience of clients.

Porous privacy sometimes takes the form of bragging – e.g., the therapist who loves to tell stories about her therapeutic triumphs. Thus, it is very important to be open about your own motivations as you look at your own behaviors. If you want something to brag about, you might want to join a bowling league or sew quilts in your spare time.

Porous privacy can also be more subtle, like simply illustrating a point with a clinical example, but with enough detail that others can tell who the person is. Or a psychotherapist might leave files and correspondence on the desk, with clients' names visible to others.

Here is a vignette for exploration:

> Chris didn't think much about the first of the following comments by his therapist, Dr Pizzarelli. But by the third one, the pattern was clear, and Chris felt he should have seen the threat to his own privacy coming.

1. Dr Pizzarelli leaned in a little toward Chris and said, "I just used this approach with another client of mine. I can't tell you who she is, but her husband was just written up in the paper yesterday for that big development project down by the river. You know the one. The big apartment complex? It was on page 1 of the business section. Had his picture and everything."

2. Patting Chris on the arm Dr Pizzarelli sounded sympathetic, "It's not unusual to feel that way. Did you see that guy who just left as you were coming in? That's Steve. He teaches chemistry at the community college. He went through the same thing about a month ago."

3. Handing Chris a card Dr Pizzarelli announced, "You mentioned last week that you were thinking about changing your life insurance. I have a friend who's a broker. When I told him about you, he said he'd be happy to help. He'll be calling you next week."

Part 1   Put yourself in the position of Chris.

- What are your reactions as you listen to Dr Pizzarelli in the first two comments?
- What are your reactions as you listen to Dr Pizzarelli in the last comment?
- Did it occur to you that Dr Pizzarelli might be mentioning you to other clients?

Part 2   Chris files a complaint with the State Regulatory Board. He charges that Dr Pizzarelli has violated the confidentiality of himself and these other clients. One of these clients also files a complaint, having heard that Dr Pizzarelli told other clients about them. The state board is charged with investigating these complaints, deciding if a violation of confidentiality has occurred and, if so, deciding on a suitable punishment or remedial plan depending on the seriousness of the violation. You are a member of the Board:

- Do you feel that confidentiality has been violated?
- On a scale from 1 to 10 with 1 being helpful and 10 being horrendous, where would you rate Dr Pizzarelli's behavior? Why?
- Was any harm done? (Refer back to the questions in Part 1.)
- What kind of discipline or punishment, if any, should Dr Pizzarelli receive?

Part 3   Put yourself in the position of Dr Pizzarelli:

- Why did you say the things you did? Think of both appropriate and inappropriate motivations.
- How could you have got the same therapeutic impact without providing information about other clients?
- What if you said the same things about a client (or conveyed the same information about a client) to a close friend over lunch, a

colleague with whom you were consulting, or a spouse as you went to bed and were sharing your day with each other?

Part 4   Finally, play with this scenario a little bit. Change the genders, ethnic backgrounds, ages, and other characteristics of the client, the psychotherapist and the Board member. Do not think only about what should happen – like ethnicity should make no difference – but what is really happening in the deepest regions of your gut.

7

Informed Consent
The Three-Legged Stool

"Knowledge is power."
Sir Francis Bacon

Our opening story comes from Mitch:

> When I was a kid, my older brother used to ask me all the time if
> I wanted to play Monopoly. And I always said, "Sure!" I was just
> learning the game, but the complexity of it intrigued me – as well,
> of course, as the thought of winning.
>
> The initial stages of the game always went quite well. I accumu-
> lated the requisite number of properties, and managed always to
> get the $10 for winning a beauty contest. But there always came a
> point in the game when my brother would introduce a new rule!
> Over time I realized that the new rules my brother introduced
> came only when I was winning, were always to my disadvantage,
> and often seemed contradictory to the new rules from our last
> game! I learned that saying "yes" to playing is not the only part of
> the game I needed to pay attention to. If I wanted to play seri-
> ously, I needed to know the rules.
>
> Within a few years I developed a reputation in my family.
> Whenever we bought a new game, I was the one who went
> through the rules before we started to play. "C'mon, Mitch!"
> they'd say as I delayed the start of many a game on a holiday
> morning. "We'll learn how to play as we go! You're holding up the
> game!" But I was not deterred. For me, knowing the rules made
> the game more fun and decreased that gnawing feeling like I was
> missing something. Even when I lost (which was frequently), at
> least I knew that I gave the game my best shot.

The Basics

Informed consent to psychotherapy is more than clients saying "Sure!" when you ask if they want to work with you as their psychotherapist. At a minimum it also involves giving clients information about the rules of the relationship, about you as a psychotherapist, and about your training – this is the "informed" part. This information is important for prospective clients to know before they say "yes."

Talking through the "rules" of the relationship is often one of the most difficult parts of therapy. Some of the rules are so complicated that it takes years for therapists to learn them accurately. Many of the rules are unique to the psychotherapy relationship; thus, clients will not just know them on their own. They need to trust us to provide enough accurate information so they know whether or not they want to enter psychotherapy with us. These are among the issues we will address in this chapter.

Informed consent may be the issue that makes the uniqueness of the therapy relationship most clear. Here's what we mean: Friends don't usually tell each other, "Listen, there's somebody on the next street that is a different kind of friend than I – perhaps you would do better with that person." Salespeople are not really obligated to tell customers that another store has a similar item that can do the job better. But in psychotherapy, therapists are obligated to tell prospective clients not only about their own therapeutic approach – risks as well as benefits – but also about other forms of help that the client may want to consider. In the words of the American Counseling Association (ACA) (2005) Ethics Code, Section A.2.a., "Clients have the freedom to choose whether to enter into or remain in a counseling relationship and need adequate information about the counseling process and the counselor."

What information do we need to give to clients? Let's take a look at two ethics codes that provide a good overview:

- NASW, 1999, #1.03: Social workers should use clear and understandable language to inform clients of the purpose of the services, risks related to the services, limits to services because of the requirements of a third-party payer, relevant costs, reasonable alternatives, clients' right to refuse or withdraw consent, and the time frame covered by the consent. Social workers should provide clients with an opportunity to ask questions.

- ACA, 2005, #A.2.b: Counselors explicitly explain to clients the nature of all services provided. They inform clients about issues such as, but not limited to, the following: the purposes, goals, techniques, procedures, limitations, potential risks, and benefits of services; the counselor's qualifications, credentials, and relevant experience; continuation of services upon the incapacitation or death of a counselor; and other pertinent information.

Think back to Mitch's story of playing Monopoly with his older brother. Some of you might have thought, "No big deal. It's just a game." You might be competitive yourself and winning is very important. For you, it seems reasonable for Mitch's brother to gain an advantage by hiding or fabricating some of the rules. Others of you might have thought, "Well, that was a crummy thing for Mitch's brother to do! What about the value of playing fair – even in a board game!"

In therapy, there is no debate about being fair or about the inappropriateness of hiding rules from clients. The therapy relationship is more like a collaborative relationship that is built upon trust. Trust can only come when the client knows the rules. In essence, the informed consent process is meant to provide enough good information to prospective clients so that they can make reasonable decisions about therapy with you. Without enough good information, prospective clients can't make an informed decision about entering psychotherapy. To get you thinking about the phrase "enough good information," take some time on the next journal entry.

Journal Entry: *Informed Consent in Our Cultures of Origin*

Part 1   Consider your college experience. Most courses had a syllabus in which the instructor outlined the "rules" for the course and other important information. In the courses you took (have taken), think about the range of information you received on the syllabi at the beginning of the term.

- How did you react to syllabi that only provided a list of dates and assignments, versus those syllabi that contained detailed information about the course, such as course goals and prerequisites?
- To the extent you wanted information, why did you want it?
- Have you had a professor change the syllabus on you?
  - How did that feel?
- Did you find that some syllabi were easier to read than others?
- If so, why?
- How might the syllabi have influenced your decisions to stay in the course, to take another course from the same professor, and to get more or less involved in the course than you would have otherwise?

Part 2   Think about some doctor visits that you have had or will have, especially when you go to the doctor for something other than a routine checkup.

- What do you want to know?
- How would you like to be told?
- What would it mean for the doctor to:
  - tell you the benefits of the treatment they are proposing?
  - tell you the risks involved? (What might *not* work in addition to what might work, and how might you be worse off if you choose the proposed treatment?)
  - tell you about other options available to help with your problem?
  - remind you of this information at various times during the course of treatment?

If the doctor did tell you about the options:

- How well did you feel like you understood the options you had?
- How comfortable did you feel with the doctor to:
  - ask questions;
  - ask follow-up questions if you didn't quite understand; and
  - refuse the treatment being offered?

The Three-Legged Stool

We refer to the informed consent process as a three-legged stool. An interesting property of three-legged stools is their stability – they do not wobble! A good informed consent process provides a stable foundation for psychotherapy. The three "legs" on which informed consent rests are ethics, law, and clinical processes. These three aspects of informed consent influence each other as we work with clients.

Ethics

Think back to the "Ten Foundations" in chapter 4. Foundation #9, "Inform clients of important information and get their consent," addresses the ethical doctrine of informing clients and getting their explicit consent to treatment. We've covered one important reason why clients need to be informed: They need to know the rules of the relationship. For example, they need to know the rules about confidentiality, the fee structure, what happens if they miss an appointment, and how they can get a hold of you in case of any emergency.

There are many other ethical justifications for the informed consent process. One justification is to think about consent in terms of clients' rights to information. In some ways, clients may be becoming better consumers of professional services. They may understand that knowledge is power and to have this knowledge they need information from the professional. They also may understand that professional relationships of any kind might work better when professionals and clients share some of the decision-making.

Foundation #9 is not the only one that speaks to the ethical justifications for informed consent. We'd like to give you an opportunity to test your sensitivity to and awareness of these issues in the next activity.

Journal Entry: *Foundations of Consent*

Look back at the ten Ethical Foundations (p. 73). Read each one of them over and think if and how each relates to possible ethical justifications for informed consent. Try to use as many Foundations as possible. Then we'll share our thoughts below.

Our Thoughts

- The most common justification for informed consent concerns respect for clients' autonomy (Foundation #3).
- Informed consent is also seen as good for treatment (beneficence, Foundation #1).
- Informed consent is a way to avoid harm (nonmaleficence, Foundation #2).
- By assuring client access good information, informed consent procedures help therapists assure fairness (justice, Foundation #4) by minimizing disadvantages some clients experience due to differences in intelligence, educational levels, cultural background, level of familiarity with psychotherapy, and other factors.

In addition to these very direct justifications, there are several indirect ethical benefits. Note these benefits below:

- By thinking about what information to provide to clients and by considering the risks and benefits of their own and others' forms of psychotherapy, therapists are helping to maintain their competence (Foundation #5).
- By providing information about the benefits of alternative methods and the risks of their own, therapists are guarding against "selling" clients on their approach (Foundation #6). (See also Red Flags: "Everybody's Everything," and "Dissing the Different;" and Green Flags: "Amicable Advice about Alternatives," "Responsible Referrals," "Informative Information," "Guarded Guarantees," and "Effective Ethical Explanations" [see chapter 4 for descriptions]).
- By clearly defining the professional relationship in an informed consent process, therapists are helping define and maintain boundaries (Foundation #7).
- If therapists take their informed consent responsibilities seriously, they are actualizing and enhancing their professional virtues such as honesty, humility, and prudence (Foundation #10).

Legal

The ethical justifications for informed consent are complemented by legal requirements about who can and cannot give consent, what kinds of information needs to be conveyed, and how much information is enough. States have laws about who can and cannot give consent. For example, children up to a certain age and legally adjudicated incompetent adults cannot give legal consent to psychotherapy. Laws set ages of consent and they differ between states. Some states require certain information to be disclosed to clients at the outset of psychotherapy so that the client or clients know what they are consenting to. In addition, some states require psychotherapists to have this information in written form called a "disclosure statement." Typically the required information is about the psychotherapist's training and some of the laws that influence the practice. For example, in Colorado psychotherapists are required to inform clients in their written disclosure statement that "in a professional relationship, sexual intimacy is never appropriate and should be reported to the board that regulates, registers, or licenses such unlicensed psychotherapist, registrant, or licensee" (CRS 12-43-214). A detailed description of legal requirements is beyond the scope of this book; however, the following references might be helpful: Appelbaum, Lidz, and Meisel, 1987; Barnett, Wise, Johnson-Greene, and Bucky, 2007.

Some therapists might be tempted to ignore their legal requirements, reasoning that if they take care of the ethical requirements they have done more than enough. This would be evidence of a separation strategy. Other therapists, perhaps adopting an assimilation strategy, might have their attorneys write their consent documents for them and ignore the ethical doctrine. An integration strategy, of course, includes both ethical sensitivity and knowledge of the law, as well as consultation with colleagues and attorneys.

Clinical

Until now you might have the impression that the requirements of informed consent represent a foreign appendage to the therapy process – a necessary but cumbersome requirement to get out of the way before therapy begins. Nothing could be further from the truth. Informed consent is part of the clinical work. Starting the therapy relationship with good information about the "rules" and respect for the client's right to refuse treatment provides a useful foundation for the working relationship (e.g., Coyne & Widiger, 1978; Jensen, Josephson, & Frey, 1989; Birch, 1990) and might actually increase the level of trust clients have for therapists (e.g., Sullivan, Martin, & Handelsman, 1993; Handelsman, 2001a). At the same time, there is wide agreement in the field that we should view consent as a *process* that happens throughout therapy, not just an *event* that occurs at the beginning (Appelbaum et al., 1987). "Informed consent is an ongoing part of the counseling process, and counselors appropriately document discussions of informed consent throughout the counseling relationship" (ACA, 2005, Section A.2.a.). It is useful to think of clients consenting to treatment every time they come to a session. The process model of informed consent can stimulate and facilitate the clinical course of therapy. For example, information about the process of therapy may stimulate clients to think about the goals of therapy and the consent can be renewed – officially or implicitly – whenever the goals of therapy evolve.

The good news is that by looking carefully at the intersection of ethical, legal, and clinical concerns, we can explore many aspects of our professional identity. At the same time, however, issues surrounding consent can cause many types of acculturation stress. Let's take a look now at the elements of informed consent and some of the acculturation tasks that are entailed.

The Culture of Consent

It is easy to say that we will give all of our clients all the information they need to make a good or informed choice about whether to see us in therapy. However, just as we learned in the last chapter about confidentiality, informed consent is multifaceted. There are several motivations and virtues we need to draw upon as we meet with new clients and help them assess the client–therapist fit.

Motivations and Virtues

Let's start with a journal entry to get you into the acculturation mood:

Journal Entry: *Personal Components of Informed Consent*

Take a look back at chapter 1 and the journal entries and food for thought items that you completed about your motivations, values, and virtues. How do these elements of your identity mesh with the justifications for informed consent we mentioned in the previous section? Do you see any situations in which you might feel a small yet strong urge to dispute or override a client's initial refusal to enter therapy with you? What information might you want to hide or share less of so that clients are more willing to work with you?

When you think about the different types of information you'll need to share during the informed consent process, write something about the feelings and reactions you might have with a client who (a) is a different gender from you; (b) is one you find very attractive; (c) appears very anxious; (d) appears very depressed; (e) has difficulty speaking English; or (f) is in some other way challenging to you.

Food for Thought: *Getting Along with a Long Consent Process*

Consider this scenario: You are seeing a new client, telling him all about your therapeutic approach and about the alternatives he may want to consider. The client seems unsure, and begins to ask lots of questions about the therapy, about you, and about other types of treatment. You cannot tell whether the client has a genuine interest in these topics or he is just "messing" with you. You find yourself getting angry and you wish he would either sign the consent-to-treatment form or just leave. What do you do? What is happening to your motivations? Are they becoming a little more varied, a little cloudier? How does the virtue of patience interact with the other virtues that you have identified as important to you as a therapist?

Here's another scenario we'd like you to write about.

Journal Entry: *Informed Refusal*

Picture this: You go through an informed consent procedure with a hypothetical client, explaining all the risks and benefits of your treatment and those of other treatments. You do a very informative job. (Think through what you would say – how you would phrase what you can offer, etc.). You know you can help the client. You are very enthusiastic and informative. As you listen to yourself you are thinking, "Wow, I have lots of excitement in my voice. I would love to work with this client and I think I am explaining my expertise well."

At the end, the client thanks you for such a clear explanation. Then she says, "Thanks, but no thanks. I'm going to pursue other options." She mentions one of the alternate treatments that you did discuss, but you know the treatment is longer and perhaps less likely to work.

- How do you feel? Are you disappointed? Are you angry or irritated? Do you feel like a failure? When clients choose to go elsewhere – especially one who has visited with us for an hour or two – at a minimum it hurts our professional pride. An experience like this can also disturb our professional myths about being helpful or about being the right therapist for every client. This type of experience may be especially hurtful when our emotional defenses are low, such as when we're experiencing problems in our personal relationships or financial problems are looming.
- What do you want to say to the client?
- Are you tempted to suggest other benefits of your approach or risks of other approaches?

- Can you respect the client's autonomy? What would make it easier to do so and what would make it harder?
- What alternatives do you have? What acculturation strategies might those alternatives represent?
- Complicating factors:
    - You need the clinical hours to graduate on time.
    - You need the money and you know money is no object for this client.
- What virtues would you like to exhibit and in what quantities?

Perspective-taking
- You have a friend who makes a similar choice not to enter therapy with a psychotherapist you think would be good, and asks your opinion of his/her decision. How do you react to your friend? What's the difference between your reactions to your client and to your friend?
- You are a client meeting a therapist for the first time. The therapist gives you a very informative picture of the benefits and risks of his approach, as well as the benefits and risks of others. As good as the presentation is, you find there's something that doesn't "click" for you with this therapist. In fact, one of the alternative approaches he talks about is new to you and sounds very interesting. You decide you'd like to give it a try. You say, "Thanks, but no thanks. I'm going to explore other options." How would you like the therapist to respond? What do you imagine is going through his head?

Not-so-simple Consent

In the example above, a client refuses treatment. A refusal makes it clear that the client does not want to work with the psychotherapist and shouldn't be forced. True consent is voluntary (Appelbaum et al., 1987). However, in some instances, the client is not voluntarily in therapy. For example, when a court orders a person to undergo treatment, the court is exercising its right to act in what it believes is the client's welfare. This is an example of paternalism. The court's judgment about the client's welfare overrides client autonomy. Indeed, it can be argued that a person under the auspices of a court does not even have autonomy to be overridden.

Another example of more complicated consent is when people are not capable of giving consent because they are not cognitively able or competent to understand enough about the situation to make a reasoned decision. One example of this is young children who are brought to treatment (either individual or family) by parents or guardians. Another example is adults who are suffering from mental disabilities. Sometimes they are adjudicated (found by a court) to be unable to give consent. Psychotherapists recognize that although a person is incompetent to give consent they should still be treated with respect by being informed about what is happening in a way they can understand. In these cases, therapists should get *consent* from parents or guardians and *assent* from the client. Several ethics codes (e.g., ACA, 2005; American Psychological Association [APA], 2002) require psychotherapists to seek assent, which means "to demonstrate agreement, when a person is otherwise not capable or competent to give formal consent (e.g., informed consent) to a counseling service or plan" (ACA, 2005, p. 20).

The application of assent may seem counterintuitive. Try this food for thought.

Food for Thought: *Assent*

Part 1 Picture this: You are a child therapist and the parents bring a 12-year-old boy for you to see. You believe you can help, the family is very motivated, but the boy is refusing to give his assent – his permission. On one hand, you'd like to honor his wish not to come. On the other hand, both you and the parents agree that even though the boy doesn't want to come, you can make therapeutic progress with him.

To give you some perspective on what this might feel like for the 12-year-old boy, consider a very common experience in the security line at the airport. You've finished going through the security door and your briefcase or backpack comes out the other side of the scanning machine.

The security agent at the station says, "May I examine the contents of your backpack?" The security person is asking for your *assent*. You can perceive this request in two ways, sometimes depending on how much of a hurry you are in: First, you can see the request as nonsensical. How crazy do you have to be to ask a question when only one answer is acceptable? After all, if you don't give assent to searching your backpack you'll have to stay home or leave your backpack here at the airport. Second, however, you can see the request as a courtesy – one step up from "Have a nice day." You and the agent both understand the situation you are in. Neither of you really enjoy the process but both are constrained to be there. Given that, it can be seen as respectful to "go through the motions."

Part 2   Consider the options you have when a client refuses to give assent: (a) You can choose not to see the client. In this case, you may not have been able to make any progress, but you may miss the chance to do some good work; (b) You can see the client in spite of their nonassent. Here, you are reversing the risks of the first option; (c) You can explore the consequences of the nonassent. Clients may not have considered the probabilities of losing services, going to jail, or continuing to be miserable with their parents; (d) You can try to compromise, perhaps having the client assent for three sessions and then reevaluate.

For each of these options, think about your possible motivations and acculturation stresses as you work with court-ordered clients and child clients, some of whom you like and some of whom you do not.

Is it just going through the motions to seek assent in therapy? Perhaps not. Some clients may not give permission and you assess that they will probably not benefit from the services you are providing. As a result, you choose not to see them. In that case, you would consult with the parents, a guardian, or the court. But don't make the "rookie mistake" of thinking that just because a court- or parent-ordered client expresses the desire not to be in therapy that nothing can be done. Good work can happen under less-than-ideal conditions. You will likely choose to see some clients who do not give you permission and, in all of these cases, it is respectful to ask the client to assent to therapy and inform him or her about what will be happening.

Information: How Much, of What Kind, Presented in What Way, Is Enough?

How do we know that a client has enough information to make a good choice about therapy without being overwhelmed by it? The question of what is enough information – and other questions surrounding informed consent – is an example of how much complexity there is behind the straightforward standard that we provide informed consent (Wise, 2007).

When dealing with informed consent in medicine, most courts adopt a "reasonable person" standard (Kitchener, 2000, p. 60) when determining how much information is enough. The question is: What would a reasonable person want to know about therapy? In Appendix A we list the types of information you might want to (or have to) disclose. We list some key areas that help clients know more about the therapeutic process, the logistics of therapy, the therapeutic process, ethical issues, and you and your training.

Green Flag: *Informative Information*

> Marvin and Clara have come to a therapist, Dr Shaw. They are having some problems with their daughter, Ashley, and these problems are either a cause or an effect of some of their marital problems. They're not sure whether they want to come as a couple, or simply to send Ashley to a therapist. After describing some of the problems, Clara asks Dr Shaw, "So tell me, Doctor: What experience do you have with issues like ours?"
>
> Dr Shaw responds, "I've had training and experience with couples, and if you want to come in for marital work I'd be happy to see you. But it's been a long time since I've seen adolescents for individual therapy, so I wouldn't feel comfortable seeing Ashley. Sometimes, it's good for a kid of Ashley's age to have her own therapist and not see her parent's therapist, anyway. If you decide to send Ashley to a therapist, I can certainly give you some names of therapists who specialize in working with adolescents."
>
> Clara says, "Well, that certainly makes our options clear." Marvin, of course, still has that 'how-much-is-this-going-to-cost-me?' look on his face.

Food for Thought: *Persuasive Information*

Think about the major approaches to therapy you have studied, including psychoanalytic therapy, cognitive behavior therapy, family therapy, existential psychotherapy, etc. For each approach: How would you describe that type of therapy to a friend of yours who may benefit from that approach, but who has not studied psychotherapy at all? Take two approaches. Can you think of ways to describe each approach that would make your friend more interested in either of them? On the flip side, can you think of ways to describe each approach that would make your friend less likely to choose either of them?

Journal Entry: *Information, Please*

Spend some time thinking about the following questions:

- What information do you *need* to convey to all clients? This information could be mandated by law, required by an ethics code or agency policy, or so basic to your work that you believe every client should know it before agreeing to come see you.
- What information might you let clients know they have a right to ask about?
- What information might you want clients to know because it will help the therapeutic process?
- On the other side of the coin, what information might you not share with clients because you believe it might actually get in the way of good work?
- What information will you disclose if asked, but only if clients bring it up? This information might be personal and/or irrelevant to therapy.

- What information would you not tell clients even if they ask?
- How do you think information and questions by clients need to be answered and in what format (e.g., oral, written)?

Acculturation Tasks and Stresses

As we mentioned before, conveying information and securing consent in psychotherapy are not analogous to many other types of relationships. Thus, part of the experience may be very uncomfortable for many therapists. Sometimes it is hard to see the informed consent process as part of the treatment process, especially when the discussion turns to risks, ethical issues, and personal information.

Therapists love to talk about the benefits, but sometimes remain silent when it comes to discussing the risks of treatment and alternative treatments. How do you feel about talking about what might go wrong? Some psychotherapists might think that talking about risks undermines the therapeutic process. Actually, predicting that rough spots are likely to come with change might have a much better effect on the therapeutic process. Remember, most clients are coming in already anxious and are likely to feel unconvinced by the message that "Everything will be fine and therapy will be smooth sailing."

Green Flag: *Amicable Advice about Alternatives*

Consider the following four responses (only the last two of which are green flags) to a client's concern:

> Chuck, 46, is facing anxieties that some people would call "midlife issues." His wife, Barbie, seems more demanding and less sexually receptive now that their nest is empty. Their son, Bill, is struggling in college, and Chuck is worried about that. At the first session with a therapist, Chuck describes these anxieties and says, "You know, I've heard that a cognitive approach works really well for these kinds of things. I'm a cognitive kind of guy. I'd really like that."

Dr Weeve: "Look, that cognitive stuff doesn't work for everybody. I think what you need is a caring, compassionate therapist, and that's what I do. I've been doing that forever. I've had lots of clients like you, who come in wanting that kind of approach and they're merely avoiding getting to the root of their existence. What they needed is what you need: a good active listener. And that's me. In fact, I had one client just about your age, who had been a high school teacher and decided to become a stock broker. Well, that was right around the tech stock bust, so he stopped that and …"

At this point, Chuck is wondering why he's getting all this detail, and why this therapist is coming down on a therapy that he's heard good things about. He thinks, "I know people who used to be high-school teachers; is she describing somebody I know [see Red Flag: Porous Privacy]? And why is she bad-mouthing a style of therapy others have found so effective [see Red Flag: Dissing the Different]?"

"… did very well. In fact, I'm seeing him on Thursday after-noons."

Chuck says, "Thank you, Dr Weeve. I'll think it over." Yeah, right.

Dr Josh Kidder: "Well, that kind of approach is pretty easy. I've taken some courses on it. I'm sure we can do that. Let's give it a try [see Red Flag: Everybody's Everything]." As Chuck leaves the office quickly, he thinks to himself, "I wonder how much training a therapist needs to be good, or even adequate, at a given kind of therapy." He decides to keep looking.

Dr Stan Tall: "I agree with you – for cognitively oriented people, it can be really great. But I'm afraid that's not my area of training. I've had a few courses, but no supervised experience. Let me give you some names of colleagues who do this kind of cognitive work [see Green Flag: Responsible Referrals]."

Dr Haive: "I see you're referred by Dr Tall; I know him. Yeah, cognitive therapy is one of my areas of expertise. My graduate advisor, Dr Welle, is a major author in that area. Let me tell you more about what I do with clients in this approach, and then you can decide if this sounds right to you. If not, I can give you names of other cognitive therapists with whom you might work better."

Red Flag: *Dissing the Different*

> During the first several minutes of her first session, Ms Valdez thought Dr Josh Kidder seemed pretty good. He was solicitous, concerned, and, although he appeared young, he was kind of cute. But Ms Valdez was still going to go through with her plan to "interview" at least two more therapists. When she mentioned this to Dr Kidder, she thought she noticed him actually flinch, as if being hit in the face with a blast of cold air. "Who are you going to see?" he asked, just a little too loud, she thought.
>
> "Well, I've heard about Dr Haive."
>
> "I can save you some time there," Dr Kidder said. "I've seen some clients who used to go to her, and they didn't have such great things to say." Ms Valdez wanted to respond that he probably saw the one or two dissatisfied clients, but wouldn't have seen any of the hundreds of satisfied customers, right? But just then, Dr Kidder said, "Who else?" a little like a prosecuting attorney.
>
> Hesitantly, Ms Valdez said, "Dr Stanley Tall."
>
> "Well, he does psychoanalytic therapy, and that can take a long time. Some people consider it just a lot of mumbo-jumbo ..." Dr Kidder waved his hand slightly in an offhand manner as his voice trailed off.
>
> "Dr Kidder, I've heard good things about these people. I'd like to check them out myself." Dr Kidder nodded and continued with the interview, but somehow he didn't seem as pleasant or as cute to Ms Valdez.

For some psychotherapists, the idea of talking about ethical issues with clients might feel uncomfortable. The discomfort might come from thinking, "If I bring these things up I'm just putting ideas into their head to see me as unethical." For example, you might be tempted to not bother the client with the details of limits to confidentiality. Your thinking might be, "Look, if I go into an oration of limits of confidentiality – about reporting child abuse and needing to protect the target of a serious threat – I am going to dissuade the client from feeling free to share anything with me. I think I am just gonna let the conversations go until I think there might be something I need to disclose." This is a potential pitfall. As we discussed in chapter 6, the client has a right to know the limits of confidentiality from the start. As with information about any issues – ethical issues, risks, etc. – if you provide such information with care and caring, the therapeutic process will be enhanced.

Food for Thought: *Credentials*

Questions about your degrees and licenses may seem like idle curiosity, but actually have a lot to do with the ethical issue of competence (Foundation #5). How do (will) you feel when clients ask you about why you are qualified to see them? Are you or will you be hesitant to answer such questions? How do you feel about clients who ask you questions that seem challenging or overly detailed? What if a client asks you for the complaint procedures of your state board?

How will you communicate your credentials? Big diplomas on the wall? Will you list memberships in professional organizations, even though they are not really indicators of competence?

The answers to these questions may give you some insight about your motivations, values, and virtues. They may also indicate particular acculturation strategies.

Perhaps the most acculturation stress comes from clients asking personal questions. Personal questions come in all shapes and sizes, ranging from those with professional aspects to very private questions. One strategy for dealing with such questions is to think about every personal question from a client as an invitation to a boundary crossing (see chapter 5, especially the section on self-disclosure). You need to think about issues such as beneficence (Foundation #1) and judge whether the answer to the question will help the client.

We might be tempted to respond fully to all requests for personal information – after all, complete honesty is a virtue, is it not? Giving into this temptation, however, would clearly be a separation strategy. In therapy – as in other relationships – honesty needs to be tempered with other virtues such as prudence and compassion.

On the other side, we might be tempted to have a policy of "no answers to personal questions." This might be evidence of an assimilation strategy, and might be too black and white – it may not give you the flexibility to make decisions based on the type of information requested, the needs of clients, their cultural identification, and other aspects of the situation.

A strategy of integration regarding personal questions involves balancing issues including honesty, prudence, beneficence, and respect. It may mean responding to clients' questions in unique and creative ways. For example: Lew and Toshiko are seeing Dr Haive for marital therapy. Just after the small talk at the first session, Lew asks with an air of politeness but an undertone of challenge: "So, are you married?" Dr Haive replies first with a simple "Yes" or "No." She then follows up with something like the following to explore the concern behind the question: "I'm wondering if you have concerns about whether I'm qualified to do couples therapy with you both?" Toshiko immediately says, "Of course we think you can!"– but with a worried look. Lew is thinking, "Damn right, I'm concerned!" but says out loud, "Well, now that you mention it …"

Another therapist might respond to the question about marriage this way: "I'm wondering whether you want to know if I've been through the kinds of problems you are going through?" This type of question is reasonable for you to ask because it shows that you are aware that all clients' questions have substance to them. Curiosity may be idle, but clients and their questions are not! The substance behind the question needs to be explored. By inviting the client to explore that substance, you as the therapist make it clear that your own personal experience is not the only, or the most basic, issue.

When Mitch was a young therapist, one question he would ask clients was, "How many couples would it take for me to have seen before you would feel comfortable?" This question made it very easy to start talking through their concerns about his competence. It also provided Mitch with the opening to make it clear that the only way to see whether he could help them is to give him a few sessions and then reassess their comfort level.

Another important acculturation task brought up by the informed consent process is to decide how collaborative the decisions about therapy are. Knowledge, as we've said, is power. Just what kind of power do clients have? Some of the information you provide to clients is clearly to educate them so they can make the decision to enter therapy or not. Clearly, they have the ultimate power and authority to make that decision. However, some information will allow clients to make other decisions that you may have thought were entirely yours. For example, you and the client may collaborate on decisions about how long to stay in therapy, what kinds of strategies (of those in which you are qualified) you will use, and how the client will be involved in their own treatment.

Red Flag: *Defensive Declarations*

> Benny, in his first session as a client, knows what probation means because he's a therapist himself. He asks Dr Weeve, "Why are you on probation with the state board?"
>
> Dr Weeve twitches noticeably before grinning widely. She says, in a voice just a little too loud, "Aaaaghh! The board was just out to get somebody to make an example of, and they came after me. That's bureaucracy for you, goin' after the little person. It's all politics."
>
> Benny thinks to himself, "This sounds like she's not taking responsibility for her actions. Does she think she's above the law? Or is she flat-out denying that she did anything wrong? Why doesn't she just tell me what she's been accused of? She could just as easily have said, 'I was found in violation of the law because I mentioned a client's name in a public place. Now, to make sure I don't mess up again, I have a supervisor.' That would have been OK."

When we think about clients needing some information from us and their possibly asking questions, the issue of *how* we answer questions becomes as important as *what* we say: One client put it this way:

> I went to see a therapist and asked some questions about his approach. He didn't answer my questions quite the way I would have liked. His approach was more laid back than I really wanted. But, you know, in answering my questions, and in exploring with me my reasoning behind the questions, I could tell that the therapist was working hard trying to understand me. He was conscientious and seemed to be a nice person. He respected my opinions, even as he explained his own point of view. I wound up seeing the therapist for a year, and I was very pleased with the results.

How we inform clients may be related to the values and virtues we hold. It is generally agreed that providing information to clients in writing is a good idea (Handelsman, 2001a), and some states require written disclosure. An even more positive approach includes giving clients a copy of the consent form (Nagy, 2000), as it increases the likelihood that clients will remember and be able to use information.

The APA (2002) code requires that the informed consent process be documented. Once again, we have several types of judgments to make, including this one:

Food for Thought: *Perspective-taking on Documentation*

Let's explore some different levels of specificity in documenting consent. Let's say you are (a) a therapist; (b) a member of an ethics committee that is investigating a therapist who is alleged to have made "guarantees of success"; or (c) a therapist (perhaps a new intern) who is taking over a case from an intern who is leaving because he has earned his degree. What level of specificity (written information) would you (a) do, (b) be looking for, and/or (c) appreciate?

- "The client signed the consent form."
- "The client and I discussed aspects of the treatment."
- "We reviewed the consent form. The client asked about the limits of confidentiality, and didn't understand at first about what 'danger to others' meant. I provided some examples of specific threats that would be reportable. The client was somewhat relieved that I wasn't going to report him just for being angry. When he signed the form, he asked for a copy before I even offered him one, and I told him that we'd go over all the information again in 5 weeks. In all the things we discussed, the client seemed most concerned about the risks of treatment I outlined – becoming more depressed, disruption in relationships, etc. Perhaps his being anxious about these things happening is related to the clinical picture of someone who is hesitant to take risks, not confident in his ability to follow through on projects, and somewhat pessimistic."

We end this chapter with a green flag story:

Green Flags: *Clear Consent and Boundary Bolstering*

Belle and Scott were upset and nervous when they came to the first session with their new therapist, Dr Kelly Verdi. After all, this was the first therapy experience either of them had ever had. Belle was feeling unsupported and wondering whether Scott might be having an affair. Scott was exasperated at being railroaded into therapy.

They were both concerned about their daughter and her weird new friends at school.

Belle and Scott were both thinking that they'd better get the first word in before their spouse contaminated Dr Verdi's judgment with false information. If they could only explain their point of view, each of them thought, Dr Verdi would surely just tell the other what they needed to do to solve the problem.

Imagine their surprise when Dr Verdi didn't let either of them speak! The first thing she did was give each of them a stack of papers. "I know this may not be what you're expecting, but we really can't begin therapy until we all agree on the ground rules. Let's go through some of the major rules together, shall we?" Dr Verdi explained that she typically sees both members of a couple but at times may want to see one individual if she thought it would help.

Belle asked, nervously, "What if Scott tells you something in secret? Are you going to keep that from me?" Dr Verdi explained that she would not keep secrets if those secrets were getting in the way of the couple treatment.

"What if I choose not to come?" Scott said, a little too angrily.

"You always have the option to terminate therapy, Scott," Dr Verdi said evenly. "Even if you decide to come for several weeks and then decide this isn't for you, you have the right to stop treatment."

"Would you still be my therapist if Scott decides he doesn't want to come in?"

Dr Verdi smiles, glad that this issue was raised so soon. "We need to talk about what your goals are, both individually and as a couple. It might be better if I work with both of you on the issues that have a direct influence on the relationship. But if you want to work on some things individually it might be a good idea for one or both of you to work with a different therapist on your own."

Belle asked, "We think our daughter may need some help; can you see her?"

"If it will help me get a sense of the family and your relationship, it might be that I'd want to see your daughter. But teenagers need somebody to talk with privately, and she may not want to open up with her parents' therapist. Again, she might do better with her own therapist."

Belle continued: "Wouldn't her therapist tell us what she was discussing?"

Dr Verdi responded, "Different therapists have different policies. When I see an adolescent in therapy I discuss with everybody, at the beginning, what kinds of information I'll convey to the parents. Usually, because I believe that kids need some privacy, I'll ask the parents to agree that I only share information when there's a clear risk to the safety of the kid."

Scott chimed in, "But the parents are paying!"

"That's right," Dr Verdi said, "and legally they have a right to the therapy information about their kid. But I ask parents to waive that right so that the kid can get the most out of therapy."

The questions and answers went on for most of that first session. There seemed to be more and more options about therapy and Belle and Scott were undecided about what to do. But Dr Verdi was in no hurry for them to make a commitment. "You need to think over what we've discussed and look over the other information I've given you," she said. "You can contact me if you decide to come in and we'll set up an appointment. If you choose not to see me, I'd be happy to give you names of other therapists who might be helpful."

At the end of the session, Belle and Scott got up slowly, as if they were both weighed down by the volume of information they had gotten and the enormity of the decisions they needed to make. But they agreed on the drive home that they felt good about Dr Verdi because she had answers to all their questions, as if she had thought about the questions beforehand. And she didn't pressure them to make a quick decision. "At least we know what we're getting into," Scott said.

"Yeah," said Belle. "Some of that stuff about us seeing other therapists would have come as quite a shock if we were three months into treatment. It's good to know this stuff now."

"Maybe we should see her for three or four sessions. Then we can have another one of these sessions where we make a final decision about who sees whom for what."

"I agree," said Belle. "That's a good idea." It was the first thing they agreed on all week.

8

Making the Most of Supervision

Here's a story from Sharon that we'll return to a bit later:

> There I was, with tears starting to form, telling my internship supervisor about my confusion in a current romantic relationship. Penny sat there listening with ears picking up on my every word and eyes intently watching my nonverbal cues. As I leaned back in my chair I thought, "How did we get onto this topic?" I remembered talking about the clients I was seeing, especially those with whom I was having some difficulty. Then I started to share some about my career goals and job application process. At that point, my thoughts got fuzzy and I began to talk about me, the person down deep inside who was trying to make sense of a conflicting personal situation. As my emotions began to unravel before Penny, she – in her gentle yet candid way – asked questions, reflected back my feelings and words, and provided some options for me to consider. Later, as I left her office and walked down the hallway to mine, I felt both clearer in my thoughts and ready for my next client of the day – one of the very clients I was having trouble with.

After reading this story, some of you might be thinking, "Wow, that was some good supervision!" Others of you might be thinking, "Wow, that was therapy when it should have been supervision!" There might be a third group of you thinking, "Wow, I don't know what that was, but it worked! It sounds like Sharon was better mentally for her next appointment, and whatever makes her ready to see clients is fine with me."

The line between therapy and supervision is just one of the complexities of supervision that we will explore in this chapter. The supervisory relationship may provoke some of the most common and acute acculturation stress for both supervisors and supervisees. After all, there is no more universal "rite of passage" for psychotherapists than supervision (Maki & Bernard, 2007), which has been described as "the critical teaching method" (Holloway, 1992, p. 177) in the helping professions. More than once we have told our students that supervision in practicum and internship can make or break the experience of entering the profession. The content and context of supervision is intricately bound up with ethics; the passing on of experience and expertise is central to the development of a "competent practitioner" (Corey, Corey, & Callanan, 2007, p. 350).

The Nature of Supervision

Supervision is a professional necessity – it is a service to the profession and the public in which a more experienced professional takes on the task of training and monitoring a less experienced professional. Although some important skills and understanding can come from books and coffee conversations, growing into a competent professional takes an intense person-to-person interaction of supervision. Maki and Bernard (2007) describe this interaction as a "mentoring/apprenticeship paradigm" (p. 348).

Supervision is a formal professional relationship. The supervisee and supervisor commit to a structure and a set of expectations and boundaries that define what will and will not happen in the relationship. Here's the way Bernard and Goodyear (2004) described the nature and goals of supervision:

> This relationship is evaluative, extends over time, and has the simultaneous purposes of enhancing the professional functioning of the more junior person(s), monitoring the quality of professional services offered to the client(s) that she, he or they see, and serving as a gatekeeper for those who are to enter the particular profession. (p. 8)

Haynes, Corey, and Moulton (2003) suggest the following four goals that supervisors need to keep in mind: (a) facilitating professional development; (b) protecting client well-being; (c) assessing the supervisee's competence and, if need be, preventing supervisees from entering the profession; and (d) helping supervisees become adept at assessing their own skill level and performance.

Before we look in detail at ethical issues inherent in supervision, we need to take stock of where you are – your ethical culture of origin – regarding some basics of supervision:

Food for Thought: *Authority Figuring*

Think about some times when you have either been evaluated (in a nonjob situation) or have needed help from somebody else regarding some skill. These times might be about tennis lessons, learning a musical instrument, or submitting drafts of your master's thesis to your advisor. They can include any time when you were facing somebody who was acknowledged as more expert than you and had some type of authority over you. As you think about these instances, explore the following questions:

1. When somebody points out a flaw in your performance, how do you react? (Did you react to this question by saying to yourself that you've never had a flaw to be pointed out?)
2. When advisors, teachers, golf pros, and other authorities make suggestions about what to do, what are your initial emotional reactions? Anger? Gratitude? Embarrassment? Joy? Sadness? (How did it feel to be behind the wheel when there was a big "Student Driver" sign on the car?)
3. Are you the type of person who likes to learn on your own or are you quick to ask for assistance? (Do you ask for directions when you are lost?)
4. When learning to master a skill, how important is it for you to appear competent even as you're learning? (When offered assistance, how quick are you to respond, "That's OK, I can do it!")

The Ethical Complexity of Supervision

The complex goals of supervision highlight a basic ethical issue: technical competence of the supervisor. Ethical and effective supervision doesn't just happen – it takes knowledge, skill, and diligence. A professional can be an ethical and effective clinician yet not a good clinical supervisor. The roles of therapist and supervisor have distinct skill sets; supervision is a specialty that requires training to develop a unique combination of "knowledge, skills, and sensitivities" (Maki & Bernard, 2007, p. 347) in areas including psychotherapy, training, and student development (Stoltenberg & Delworth, 1987).

Journal Entry: *Acculturation to Supervision – the Good, the Bad, and the Beautiful*

This exercise builds on what you've learned in the last exercise: Think of a time when you were supervised in a job or task. It could be with a psychotherapy supervisor or any kind of structured job supervision. Now that you have that in your mind, write down responses to the following questions:

1. What happened in that supervision that prompted you to grow and develop?
2. What happened in that supervision that hindered you from growing and developing?
3. How did you contribute to the good outcomes?
4. How did you contribute to the bad outcomes?
5. If you erred in some way, which way was it and why – e.g., wanting to do things your own way, not taking enough initiative and simply doing what you were told, or just doing the minimum required?

The ethics codes of the major psychotherapy professions all have some things to say about supervision, including prohibitions against sex and other multiple relationships with supervisees, maintaining competence, and respecting confidentiality. Some states now require people who want to be supervisors to take special training and secure specific credentialing in clinical supervision before they can provide supervision.

Rather than simply review the rules around ethical supervision, we want to take a more comprehensive and positive approach. Our starting point is to recognize the complex roles of both supervisors and supervisees and to assert that engaging in supervision is itself an act of moral courage! Supervisors are ethically and legally responsible for their supervisees' choices and behaviors (Harrar, VandeCreek, & Knapp, 1990). This is a significant obligation and a prime example of possible acculturation stress for supervisors. They must continually balance the needs of many people and entities, including trainees, clients, agencies, state regulatory bodies, and their own selves.

As supervisors, we try to balance the obligation of our gatekeeping role – keeping some trainees *out* of the profession – with attempting to maintain a supportive atmosphere, which is conducive to good supervision (Carifio & Hess, 1987; Wulf & Nelson, 2000; Martino, 2001). We try to achieve this balance by being very clear about our goals with supervisees. For example, in Sharon's ethics class and then in the teaching/ supervising practicum, she shares two very important messages with her students. The first message is that as their supervisor she always wants them to know that her supervision is characterized by concurrent and appropriate levels of both support and challenge. The support part is about Sharon providing an environment where supervisees experience a safe place to be honest and accountable about their work with clients. The challenge part is about her assessing their skill level and ability to ensure that their clients are receiving the best possible service. Her goal is that trainees continue to grow and develop as competent, ethical counselors.

Sharon's second message to her students and supervisees may be perceived either as a harsh reality or as a shared superordinate value: Although Sharon cares about her trainees and their professional development, she makes it clear that her greater obligation of care is for their clients. For example, if a supervisee is impaired and clients are not being well served, it is her ethical obligation to the student and to the profession to address the issue. If need be, she will shut the gate to keep a student from entering into the profession. As Barnett, Erickson Cornish, Goodyear, and Lichtenberg (2007) discuss, the role of gatekeeper has received limited press, yet is a vital part of the supervisor's responsibilities. Although this isn't the most pleasant of issues to present to students, it needs to be explicitly recognized, and being honest and direct with students is another superordinate value.

Supervisees have balancing acts as well. For example, they have to balance their interests in appearing competent to their supervisor with being humble and honest in supervision so they can learn as much as possible. In other words, supervisees need to embrace supervision that both supports and challenges them. When supervisors create a safe supervision relationship, supervisees can feel freer to share their work openly and more effectively (Barnett, Erickson Cornish et al., 2007). They can seek and accept critical feedback and develop the ability to benefit from increasing levels of challenge. One integration strategy might be to replace the value of looking competent *as a therapist* with the value of being *effective and competent as a trainee*! Being an effective trainee includes making errors, sharing uncertainty, self-reflection, and being able to learn from these experiences.

These multiple balancing acts can be a primary source of stress and make supervision one of the more difficult, taxing, and ethically challenging aspects of the psychotherapy profession. Sherry (1991) discusses three factors that make supervision difficult and supervisors "vulnerable to misconduct" (p. 568). First, there are competing or conflicting role obligations, especially for the supervisor. Second, the supervision hour can feel "therapy-like." Third, there is a power differential between the supervisor and supervisee. Let's explore each of these three factors.

Role Obligations

We've already touched on the constant tension among supervisors' role obligations: How do supervisors help supervisees develop their skills and be appropriately challenged while assuring an adequate level of service to clients? Let's think about these roles some more:

Food for Thought: *Your Favorite Student*

Imagine that you are on the part-time faculty of a training program and that part of your work is being a supervisor. Your favorite supervisee, Sue, is just finishing up her practicum before going on internship. Late in the semester during one of your supervision sessions, Sue casually mentions that she has routinely been meeting clients for coffee. When you ask how long this has been going on, she says, "I've always done this with a few of my clients whom I feel benefit from the more informal interactions."

"Why haven't you told me this before?" you ask.

"It's not like a date or that I'm having sex with any of these clients; it's always been in the interest of the therapy. I didn't think it was important to mention it."

Sue clearly has not learned the lessons of her training program (including those in chapter 5). What she has done is clearly unethical (although you still have lots of information to get), and is grounds for a dismissal hearing in front of the program ethics committee. If Sue is found guilty of unethical behavior (which she surely would be), the committee has several options: they could discharge her from the program, delay her internship for a year, fail her in her practicum, or put a letter of admonition in her file. How do you react?

- Do you file the case with the ethics committee?
- Do you have a "heart-to-heart" conversation with Sue, letting her know that what she has done is serious enough to warrant an ethics committee investigation?
- Do you consider her stellar academic record and decide to let this go if she promises to tell you absolutely everything she's doing in therapy from now on?

The program policy clearly states that "all serious ethical infractions by students need to come to the attention of the program." As you're thinking this over, consider the following questions:

1. Which of these statements are you most tempted to say or think?
    a. "I know it's program policy, but this can be handled much more effectively in the context of our supervision. After all, I've been Sue's supervisor for a long time and I know her well."
    b. "I've got to turn this into the ethics committee. What will they think of me if I don't?"
    c. "This program has too many rules for students to follow. I am not going to turn this into a big deal."
    d. "This is an uncomfortable situation. I really value Sue's work and she's done a good job. This misstep is serious, though. I think I need to bring this up with the faculty and discuss our possible steps of action."
2. Which acculturation strategies might these statements represent?
3. *If you are leaning toward turning her in:* Several of the senior ethics committee members have been complaining about their responsibilities lately, stating that they think professors have been too quick to forward to the committee cases that should be handled between the supervisor and supervisee. If you turn Sue in, you wonder how that will affect your reappointment to your faculty position next year (i.e., you want to keep your job). Will this rock the boat?
4. *If you are leaning toward handling Sue yourself:* Several of the senior ethics committee members have been complaining about their responsibilities lately, stating that they think professors have not been forwarding cases to the committee that are too serious to be handled in supervision. If you handle the situation yourself, you wonder how that will affect your reappointment. You really don't want to rock the boat.
5. How would your reactions change under the following conditions?
    a. Sue was an international student from Kenya.
    b. It was Sue's first semester in the program, rather than last.
    c. Sue was a marginal student and not your favorite.
    d. Sue asked you to keep this from her major professor, who would "have my behind" if he found out.
    e. Sue was Sam.
    f. Sue had only gone for coffee once, with one client, after she had successfully terminated therapy.
    g. Upon further investigation you find that she only went for coffee with clients who were attractive single males.

Food for Thought: *Your Favorite Supervisor*

Put yourself in the place of a trainee. You are talking to one of your fellow trainees about a particularly difficult and distasteful client you have and you inadvertently mention his name. Your colleague says, "That's my cousin!" You apologize profusely to your colleague, and extract from him a promise not to turn you in for your breach of ethics, assuring him that you will tell your supervisor.

As your meeting with the supervisor looms closer and closer, your thoughts wander to several different options. First, you consider the possibility that it would be respectful to your client if you told him about the breach of confidentiality and apologized to him. You wonder what your supervisor (whom you really like and trust) would say about that. Then you think, no harm was actually done to the client and he doesn't need to know of the breach. And then there is the good impression you have been making on your supervisor recently and the letter of recommendation she has promised to write for you.

1. Consider the following possible steps:
   a. You choose to tell your supervisor about your behavior. Why?
   b. You choose not to tell your supervisor about your behavior. Why?
2. How do your reasons fit with the values and virtues in your journal?

Now, imagine that you do tell your supervisor, who thinks it over and then says to you, "What you just told me is a serious ethical infraction. I'm afraid I need to refer your case to the program's ethics committee. The consequences might be very severe." Which of the following is closest to your reaction?

1. "I deserve to be kicked out of the program. That was an unacceptable ethical error."
2. "I made a mistake. I'll address the ethics committee as best as I can and learn from the situation. I'll ask for a second chance."

3. "Mentioning a client's name is no big deal. My supervisor is way too harsh."

Which acculturation strategies might these statements represent?

Think about what facts would need to change for your reactions – and your acculturation strategies – to be different.

The Therapy-like Feel of Supervision: Boundary Issues and Beyond

In some ways, supervision is – or at least appears to be – similar to psychotherapy. For example, one person comes to another for help; the professional relationship is a key to the success of the enterprise; and there is power to be used, shared, and potentially exploited. But supervision is a unique relationship and very different from a therapy relationship. One difference is the focus of concern and welfare. For therapists, the concern for clients' welfare is paramount. For supervisors, the concern is for the supervisees' development *in addition to* clients' welfare.

A second difference is that supervisees have ethical obligations in a supervisory and therapeutic relationship that clients do not have in the professional relationship. For example, supervisees need to be honest, self-reflective, prudent, and humble with their supervisor. Supervisees also have obligations to their clients to be competent, truthful, and concerned about client welfare. Clients, on the other hand, aren't obligated to demonstrate these same attributes.

Parallel process is one of the most interesting phenomena we encounter in supervision. More times than we can count, an experience is happening in supervision between us and our supervisee that is similar – in an important way – to what is happening in therapy between the supervisee and client. For example, there have been times when our supervisees felt frustrated with us when we've asked questions (rather than gave answers) which is similar to the client's response when our supervisee asks questions rather than giving answers to the client. In each case, the person frustrated just wants "the answers." There have also been times when what is happening in the client's life has a similar ring to what is happening in the supervisee's life – which can be another type of parallel process. Understanding parallel process can give us insight not only into our clients' behaviors, but into our own behaviors, motivations, and needs both as supervisors and supervisees. This takes us back to the opening story of the chapter.

Food for Thought: *Therapy or Supervision?*

Reread Sharon's story at the beginning of this chapter. Consider the following questions:

1. What was your first impression of what occurred? Did it sound like supervision or did it sound like therapy?
2. If you are not sure, what else would you want to know to make a decision? In other words, what distinguishes therapy from supervision?
3. As a supervisor, how much personal information might you want to know about your supervisee's life in order to know how you might best help them develop?
4. As a supervisee, what type of questions from your supervisor might you find intrusive and prefer not to answer?
5. As a supervisee, what type of questions from your supervisor might you find helpful and wish to answer?
6. Have you had a similar experience in a supervision session? If so, what did it feel like to you?
7. Reflect on the different issues we've explored thus far and see which ones relate to Penny (the supervisor) and which ones relate Sharon (the supervisee).

The sometimes fluid boundary between therapy and supervision brings up other boundary considerations. Think about the issues we discussed in chapter 5; many of them can be applied here. Consider, for example, the supervisor who engages in inappropriate self-disclosure during supervisions sessions, or brings their personal problems into the sessions, or shows bias or discrimination against supervisees based on supervisee's personal beliefs or lifestyle (Cornish, Kitchener, & Barnett, 2008). In a parallel way, think about a *supervisee* who engages in inappropriate self-disclosure (during therapy or supervision), brings their personal problems into sessions, or shows bias or discrimination against clients.

Negotiating boundaries might be more difficult in supervision than in therapy because the differences between supervisees and supervisors may be less salient than those between clients and therapists or students and professors. For example, both supervisees and supervisors are professionals in the same field, they are both there to discuss the problems of the client, and they might be closer in age than the client and therapist. Thus, the illusion might be that boundaries can be more fluid in supervision. However, we take a similar position as in chapter 5 regarding boundaries between therapists and clients. That is, we believe that keeping boundaries "pure" and as free as possible from competing obligations and conflicts of interest serves everyone best.

Food for Thought: *Boundaries*

Scenario 1   Sarah, a first-year professor in the graduate program, thought that her supervision with a first-year student, Arturo, had been unusually intense but unusually productive. Arturo was the first person in his family to go to college, let alone graduate school. Many of the supervision sessions consisted primarily of Sarah sharing her "wisdom" about academia with him; after all, she had landed this plum job only six months ago. In these sessions, Arturo had talked a lot about his own feelings of intimidation and his fears of not doing well. Arturo had done well with his clients and asked that Sarah be his supervisor for the next semester. Sarah accepted the invitation and looked forward to working with Arturo again.

One day while she and Arturo were talking in her office, Sarah gets the call she'd been waiting for: a summer position at a research lab on the coast! She tells Arturo, who shares her excitement. Before Sarah realizes what she is doing, she asks Arturo, "Would you like to house-sit my house this summer?"

Scenario 2 Susan appreciated the way Krisann worked with clients, especially children. On several occasions Krisann found a way to connect with even the most reserved and reticent child. For sure, Krisann was one of the best psychotherapists-in-training that Susan had worked with. Krisann was graduating in the summer and Susan was pleased to write a letter of recommendation.

At their last supervision session for the term, Susan and Krisann briefly shared their plans for the summer. When Krisann found out that Susan and her husband were taking a short vacation and needed child care, Krisann quickly volunteered, "I would love to babysit your kids!" At first, Susan felt relief. She believed Krisann would be a great and trustworthy sitter for her children. And of the few sitters she trusted and typically employed, none of them were available for that long weekend. But then Susan felt uneasy. She felt like this could be a problem of role confusion. So, she said, "Thanks for the offer, Krisann, but I think it's probably best if I don't hire a student to babysit my children."

Look back to chapter 5 and respond to the following questions:

1. Are there potential boundary crossings or violations in these situations?
2. Do any of the Green Flags or Red Flags apply here? If so, which ones, and how?
3. If you were Arturo or Krisann, what would you be thinking?
4. If you were another student who heard about this offer from Sarah to Arturo or the offer from Krisann to Susan, what would you be thinking?
5. What factors or changes in the scenarios might make this situation either more or less serious?
6. If you were on an ethics committee and were considering a complaint against Sarah in Scenario 1, what might you be thinking?

Power Differential

Although the differences in roles between supervisor and supervisee sometimes seem much less salient than those in other professional relationships, the stakes are very high and there is a strong power differential. Much of the power derives from the evaluation and gate-keeper roles that supervisors play. Of course, properly balanced and judiciously applied power can be of benefit to both supervisees and their clients.

What might the *misuse* of power look like? Once again we can draw parallels from the therapy relationship. One misuse might be indoctri-nation. By this we mean that supervisors squelch supervisees' profes-sional growth by limiting their ways of working with clients to how the supervisors would do it. This would be parallel to therapists advising clients to solve problems the way the therapists have, even though clients have other resources to use. Another misuse of power is the imposition of personal values that negatively influence supervisees' work with clients. For example, supervisors might value a pro-choice or pro-life position and encourage trainees to nudge the client in a direction that matches the supervisors' value set.

Making the Most of Supervision

The professional literature suggests that the relationship between the supervisor and supervisee is the most important part of supervision (Loganbill, Hardy, & Delworth, 1983; Barnett, Erickson Cornish et al., 2007). A healthy, functional relationship is one free of power struggles and replete with healthy doses of virtues on the part of both parties. The supervisee needs to experience the supervisor as empathic, respect-ful, supportive, and committed to or emotionally invested in the supervisee's development (Kennard, Stewart, & Gluck, 1987; Watkins, 1995). Both parties need to experience the other as trustworthy and collaborative in the relationship (Ellis, 1991; Henderson, Cawyer, & Watkins, 1999; Ladany, Ellis, & Friedlander, 1999; Wulf & Nelson, 2000).

Virtues

We see several virtues as being key to a productive supervision rela-tionship. The first is honesty. Supervisors need to give honest feedback about how supervisees are performing in their role as psychotherapists. Supervisees need to give honest information about how therapy is pro-gressing and how they are experiencing supervision.

Remember in chapter 1 when Sharon shared her supervision experience? Her professional ego got pinched when her internship supervisor pointed out her missteps with a couple and even highlighted her colluding with the wife's verbal harshness in the relationship. Her supervisor's honesty did hurt, but because it was tempered with virtues like compassion it obviously had an impact, seeing as how she can remember the conversation so many years later. The second part of that story (and the part she likes to remember the most) is that in her next session she corrected the situation directly with the clients. She shared with them her supervisor's observation and apologized to the husband for not really hearing him. The therapeutic work then continued on a better track.

Honesty also refers to honesty with oneself. Supervisors need to be honest about their interests, their personal and professional reactions to supervisees, and their motivations. Supervisees need to be honest about their own motivations, strengths, weaknesses, and reactions. When honesty is a norm of the relationship, each party can be real and feedback can be more effective.

Being real and honest in the supervisory relationship leads to a second important virtue: humility. For example, supervisors need to be clear about the limits of their competence and not promise supervision in an area that goes beyond their scope of practice. Supervisees need to be willing to receive negative as well as positive feedback about their work and embrace the guidance given to make course corrections.

Third, humor is important, especially when it is used in combination with humility and honesty. Being willing to laugh at yourself and sharing the funny situations are healthy dynamics in the supervisory relationship. They allow us to gain perspective. For example, when supervisors share their human foibles, supervisees can relax a bit and come to see that being a "good therapist" does not translate into being a "perfect therapist."

This is only a partial list of necessary virtues. Look back to your own list and see how your virtues – the ones you have and the ones you need to develop – apply on both sides of the supervision relationship.

Informed Consent

In the previous chapter we talked about informed consent with clients. Similar to therapy, the supervisor/supervisee relationship is a contractual one (Sherry, 1991) that benefits from an informed consent process to spell out the expectations and obligations involved (Bernard & Goodyear, 2004). As we mentioned before, supervision is a critical part of the psychotherapist's development. The task is to have a good match between supervisor and supervisee, and, as we said in chapter 7, to have both parties clear on the "rules of the game."

What information might be exchanged? As a supervisee, you certainly have the right to know how and when you will be evaluated by the supervisor. You also have the right to know what is expected of you for each supervision session. Do you bring audiotapes or videotapes of sessions? Do you bring all of your case notes for the supervisor to read, or just summary notes? On the other side of the relationship, supervisors need to clarify several issues. For example, we need to describe how supervision will work and our philosophy of supervision. We also need to let supervisees know if there's a fee for supervision, and how we will be available to supervisees if and when there is an emergency.

Food for Thought: *Informed Consent and Supervision*

Look back to chapter 7 and consider the parallels between supervision and therapy. From the supervisee's perspective, ask yourself: What other information would you like to know about supervision and your supervisor? Then, from the supervisor's perspective, ask yourself: What would you want a supervisee to know before they choose to work with you?

When Things Go Wrong

Unfortunately, it is not rare that some degree of conflict occurs in supervision (Baird, 1999). Reasons for such conflict include personality clashes, supervisory style, and differences in theoretical orientation.

When conflicts occur, there are several steps to take and issues to consider (Baird, 1999). First, look at the problem or conflict as an opportunity to learn something about yourself – look for that nugget of gold. Second, try to identify what the conflict is about. In other words, get clear in your own mind how you see the conflict before you discuss it with your supervisor. After you have identified what you believe the conflict to be about, ask yourself, "What part of this conflict am I responsible for? What principles or virtues are at stake? How am I willing to change?" Third, try to see the issue from your supervisor's point of view if you can. Perspective-taking is an important element in any human relationship.

As a supervisee you have a difficult problem on your hands when the supervision you are getting is poor. The supervisor could be technically incompetent, due to bad training, temporary impairment, or other reasons. The supervisor might also be acting unethically. Confronting a supervisor can be a difficult process. You need to decide, for example, whether the problem you are seeing might be something *you* are doing, like being resistant to good ideas. If you decide that the supervisor does have a problem that results in bad or unethical supervision, confronting the supervisor takes moral courage.

Another consideration when you face an issue regarding an unethical or incompetent supervisor is to seek out support. This support might be from another professional, a faculty member at your program, your own therapist, and/or a family member.

Sometimes it's hard to talk with other faculty members: We have seen students go through a whole semester of poor supervision, not saying anything to us or other faculty. The student's thinking was either, "I can't tell anybody because I'll be seen as a poor student" or, "I am probably just overreacting and I can get through this on my own." Students often suffer alone in bad supervision when at a minimum they could have shared their burden with other faculty members and likely have got some support.

A Word about Consultation

Although the skills and activities involved in consultation are similar to those in supervision, there are differences. Here are two major differences: First, consultation is between two peers. Supervision is between an experienced professional and a less experienced professional. Second, the consultant is expected to give good professional advice and direction to the person seeking consultation; however, there is no legal liability or ethical liability on the part of the consultant. But remember, in supervision, the supervisor is ethically and legally responsible for the professional practice and choices of the supervisee.

Here's an interesting reality: You'll never be too experienced or too much of an expert not to need some guidance! Consultation is a wonderful gift to give and receive. Although the ethical pitfalls might be less severe because the power differential is smaller and there is no evaluative component to the relationship, it is still important to maximize the benefit you get from consultation. We have a few suggestions for you about how to choose a consultant.

Our first suggestion is to remain humble enough to ask for help when you need it. Second, consider whether you want clinical or ethics consultation. Although in both cases you want to look for experts, we feel that ethics consultation may take a little more prudence as you select a consultant. For example, when choosing a clinical supervisor, you might want to find someone who is more expert than you in your own form of therapy. However, if you need ethics consultation, it might be more prudent to choose a consultant who is expert in ethics but who does *not* work with clients from the same theoretical orientation! This will give your discussions more perspective.

Third, do not consult with colleagues who are your friends! Again, this is especially true for ethics consultation – you do not want to put friends or close colleagues into the awkward position of having to give you bad news about your ethical behavior.

Fourth, make consultation routine. Set up regular consultation with a group of professionals who commit to being honest with each other and call for accountability among the group members.

Finally, we feel that the more serious the problems you are having, either clinical or ethical, with the case the more formal you want the consultation relationship to be. This means you should begin the relationship with an informed consent process. Document the consultation. Pay for it. This will help you take it seriously and get the perspective and guidance you need.

Green Flag: *Beneficial Boundary Bolstering*

Dr Newman hadn't been in practice long when she realized that the world is more complex than the academy! She knew all the platitudes about "Put your client's needs first," "Provide enough information so your clients can make good decisions," and "Don't exploit your clients financially." But putting these into practice with a wide range of clients was a daunting task. Dr Newman decided to hire an ethics consultant who could look over what she was doing and suggest some ways to make what she considered an ethical practice even better.

The first person she thought of as a consultant was her old ethics teacher, Professor Sandoval. He knew her well, and he always told his students, "Let me know if you have questions."

When Prof. Sandoval heard from Dr Newman, one of his best students of the last few years, he was delighted. It made his heart feel good to know that his students had learned the lessons he tried to teach, including the value of thinking about ethics and the ongoing nature of ethical development. When she asked to see him as a consultant, however, Prof. Sandoval needed to teach one more lesson.

"I'm not the person you want for this," he started.

"But ... but ... you said we could contact you with questions. You wrote that wonderful letter of recommendation for my internship and my first job! You said I was one of your best students."

"That's *exactly* why I'm not the best person to give you consultation. I'm biased, if only slightly, and my interests are conflicted. You need a consultant who can be objective and honest. I think I could be honest, but it might be hard for me to tell you that what you are doing is not good."

"But I just need somebody to look at what I'm doing in case ..." Dr Newman trailed off, as if she had just started to realize what Prof. Sandoval was about to say.

"Yeah, but think of a situation in which you get complained against," Professor Sandoval said, picking up on Dr Newman's growing insight. "What would an ethics committee say when you told them that you got consultation from your old professor, a colleague who was already favorably predisposed toward you and might see your behavior as a reflective of *his own* professional effectiveness? How objective is that going to look? I can give you names of a few folks whom you don't know who can offer you a more objective view."

"I see what you mean," Dr Newman replied. After she got the names from him and thanked him, she hung up the phone and immediately decided to increase her annual donation to her school's alumni association …

9

Ending Psychotherapy
The Good, the Bad, and the Ethical

"Parting is such sweet sorrow."
William Shakespeare

As we (Sharon and Mitch) write this penultimate chapter, we are nearing the completion of a six-year process. Most of the rest of the book has been written, and the end is in sight – in fact, we're facing a looming deadline. Here's our question: When will we know that the book is good enough to publish – when is it actually finished? We have been discussing both substantive and process issues for years, and the questions keep on coming: Do we have enough journal entries in each chapter? Does our discussion of boundaries lean too heavily on our own values, or not enough? Are we being too prescriptive on the chapter on informed consent? Should we say more about giving advice in therapy, or is that not enough of an ethical issue? Are we positive enough in our approach? Have we really got our important points across to help readers with their ethical acculturation?

How do we know when we have put in enough effort, with enough impact, to produce an optimal outcome? At what point is a substandard product so bad that we are displaying incompetence? At what point would more polishing of the manuscript be evidence of our own fear rather than our desire, and ethical obligation, to help our readers? We can never have perfect answers to these types of questions; we would need *infinite* time and *infinite* judgment. However, if we used this lack of perfection as an excuse and chose to totally ignore these types of questions, the manuscript may turn out to be of little value.

In therapy, the same types of questions arise: "Is therapy done? Have we done all that we can do for right now?" However, you might be saying to yourself: The questions about ending therapy are much easier because I have the client right there. All I need to do is ask. Why is there an entire chapter just on termination? Most ethics books don't empha-size the issue of termination; however, the ethics codes declare the importance of this part of therapy. For example:

- AAMFT, 2001, #1.9: Marriage and family therapists continue therapeutic relationships only so long as it is reasonably clear that clients are benefiting from the relationship.
- NASW, 1999, #1.16: (a) Social workers should terminate services to clients and professional relationships with them when such services and relationships are no longer required or no longer serve the clients' needs or interests.

These guidelines seem to be straightforward and to the point. Seems pretty simple – all we need to add is the idea that clients are free to terminate and we're covered, right?

Almost! The platitudes about termination – the client has the choice of when to terminate, therapists should terminate when therapy isn't working any more – are not so easy to implement, for two reasons. First, the platitudes and principles often conflict with each other. Second, terminations involve difficult clinical judgments, complex personal reactions, and challenges to many of our virtues. Here's a related example: When we finish writing this book, we will feel elated, relieved, and probably quite successful. Six years of hard work will have paid off, our professional identities as educators will have been bolstered, and our values of achievement and industry will have been actualized. However, we will experience other reactions as well: We will feel scared that we've missed something, or that we could have anticipated the needs of a wider spectrum of our readers. We will feel sad to lose the opportunity to work with each other. We may even feel terrified at having to face the void left by the completion of our task – what do we do now?

In a similar way, psychotherapy termination always means a complex set of reactions that are related to your ethical acculturation. Thus, our goal in this chapter is to explore your ethical acculturation in regard to termination by looking at some positive elements of the process and some ethical and acculturation choices around two basic questions: When should termination of psychotherapy happen? And, who decides when to terminate, client or therapist? Let us start with some self-exploration.

Journal Entry: *Endings*

How are you at ending relationships? What do you experience and how do you navigate them? Think about several different types of relationships you've had that have ended, including (but not limited to) some of the following:

- romantic relationships;
- close friendships that ended when you graduated or moved away;
- roommates;
- relationships with co-workers, employers, or employees.

Think about relationships that have ended because: (a) you initiated the termination (breakup, move, etc.); (b) the other person initiated the termination; and/or (c) the ending came about because of external circumstances. Think about endings that were good and those that weren't so good. Think about endings that you've regretted. Now, reflect in writing about questions such as:

- How did (do) you feel at the end of these relationships?
- What is your typical pattern with ending relationships before they need to be ended? For example, are you more likely to quit before you get fired or do you hang on to the relationship even when the "writing is on the wall"?
- What types of relationships and what types of endings are relatively easy for you and which are harder?
- When endings are difficult, to what extent do you look for internal guidance (go with your feelings), and to what extent do you look for external sources of help (e.g., saying things like, "Our policy is such that …")?
- Do you "walk away," or are you the type of person who likes to "process" the end – to look back and reflect on what the ending means?
- How else might you characterize what you think, feel, and do at the end of different types of relationships?

The Good and the Ethical: Positive Elements of Termination

One positive way to think about termination is that it is the logical conclusion to the ongoing informed consent process that occurs during therapy. It may be the time that the client, with full information, finally chooses to say, "I'm done." Indeed, some authors have encouraged therapists to cover the issue of termination during the initial consent process (Kramer, 1986). Rice and Follette (2003) advise therapists to "take responsibility at the beginning of a therapy contract for educating the client on how the termination process will unfold and what criteria you will be using to evaluate their progress" (p. 157). All relationships end and explicitly acknowledging this fact at the beginning of a therapeutic relationship provides useful information for both therapists and clients.

Both the APA (2002) and ACA (2005) codes mention *pretermination counseling*. For example, the ACA code states that "counselors provide pretermination counseling and recommend other service providers when necessary" (2005; A.11.c.). Pretermination counseling can be viewed as providing information so clients can make an informed refusal and, similarly to the informed consent process at the beginning of therapy, get information about other sources of help. Even when therapy ends well, you and your client can take some time to recap your work and the therapeutic relationship, talk some about how it feels, and say goodbye. Of course, sometimes clients drop out of therapy before any pretermination counseling can be done.

We'll talk later in the chapter about how you might provide some pretermination information in the most ethical way. For now, we turn our attention to some difficult ethical decisions you will need to make in every therapeutic relationship you have. We've organized this discussion around two basic and practical questions. These questions will help you navigate the ethical landscape and integrate your values and virtues from your ethical cultures of origin, the tendencies about endings that you identified in your journal entry, and professional standards and principles. The questions revolve around when therapy should end and who decides.

When Should Psychotherapy End?

The best-case scenario is when you and your client agree on when therapy is over. Sometimes, however, you and the client have different ideas about whether this is the end, and sometimes the answer isn't even clear to you. We assume that the decision about when therapy is over can be very emotional for clients. We need also to remember that it can be just as emotional for us because it involves our personal and professional values, clinical judgment, and therapeutic orientation.

Let's assume for the moment that there is an objectively and determinable perfect time for any therapy to end. At the risk of sounding like Goldilocks, we can look at termination along a continuum: it can be too soon, too late, or just right. When we say "too soon" or "too late," we are not talking about a matter of minutes, hours, or days; even weeks might still be within ethical limits. After all, physicians are not always sure of the exact time when a cast should come off or a medication discontinued. At some point, however, rushing or delaying termination goes beyond acceptable judgment, perhaps beyond poor judgment. It can move to a situation in which clients do not benefit as much as they could have or in which they are harmed.

The ethical components of deciding when therapy is over include several factors, including these: having the clinical competence to assess the (lack of) progress of therapy, the virtues of prudence and humility which allow us to make that determination without our personal needs getting involved, and to actualize our professional values regarding such issues as what therapy is for and what it means for particular clients.

One condition under the "just right" part of the continuum is for all the client's problems to be solved. Another condition is that the results of the therapy are *good enough*. In these scenarios, not all the client's problems have been solved, but enough have been resolved so that the client feels ready – at least for some period of time – to walk through life without your guidance and support. A third condition is that therapy did not work well enough to continue. A fourth condition is that therapy didn't work at all, and a fifth, that therapy actually harmed the client.

Food for Thought: *Is Therapy Over?*

Take a look at the following vignettes and ask yourself if these are satisfactory outcomes and whether therapy should end. And why or why not? Think of each vignette from the perspectives of (a) the therapist, (b) the client, and (c) a supervisor. Think about what you would do, or what you would encourage a supervisee to do – and why – from an ethical perspective. Also consider what might be evidence of acculturation strategies of integration, assimilation, and separation.

- A client comes in to stop smoking and seven weeks later has kicked the habit. However, now he's feeling some sadness.
- A woman comes in feeling depressed. Seven months later she is feeling much better – taking much more control of her life. She still reports times of sadness that last for long periods, but she is able to go about her life; e.g., she always manages to get to work.
- A couple comes in for counseling and their stated goal is to save the relationship. After 14 long months they agree to stay together. From your perspective it seems like one partner is getting the "better deal" and is more comfortable with the outcome than the other.
- A couple comes in for counseling. Their goal was to try and keep the relationship together – for the sake of the kids. After 14 stormy months they decide to get divorced. Neither partner is happy, but they seem resigned to their decision and they both talk about looking forward to what the future brings.

You might still be thinking, "OK, I hear what you are saying but this really seems pretty straightforward." But sometimes therapists and/or clients get into a rut – it just feels good to be in psychotherapy and neither party questions the weekly appointments. However, convenience or habit is not enough to justify continued treatment. Therapists shouldn't keep seeing clients because they get used to seeing them and have nothing else to do on Tuesday afternoons. And clients should not come to therapy just because it passes the time pleasantly, or because they enjoy visiting with the therapist, or because it's a good way to avoid making friends. None of these are good reasons to continue therapy.

Who Initiates the Discussion of Termination?

Let's expand our discussion by adding another dimension to the mix – who decides to end treatment, or who initiates the discussion. Below in Figure 9.1 is our complete graphic showing both continua.

Clients can initiate a discussion of termination – or, of course they can simply leave and not come back. Therapists can initiate the discussion and in some cases unilaterally decide to end treatment. Or the termination can be a truly collaborative effort. The best-case scenario is the latter where both you and your client feel like the contract has been met. Alternatively, both you and your client may agree that therapy has *not* been helpful and is not likely to be. In either situation there is a perfect intersection of beneficence and client autonomy: what's best for the client in your judgment is also what the client is choosing.

Of course, relatively few therapies end right at the middle of our diagram in Figure 9.1. We are more likely to find ourselves in one of the other boxes in our figure, which represent unclear or conflicting answers to the questions of providing benefit and respecting client choice. Let's explore the top row first, in which therapists initiate termination.

When to Terminate

		Too Soon	Just Right	Too Late
Who Decides?	Primarily the Therapist	[abandonment]		
	Both Therapist and Client		[perfection!]	
	Primarily the Client			[dependence]

Figure 9.1 A matrix for termination decisions

Therapist-initiated Termination that's Just Right

In spite of the adage that clients are in control of the decision to come for therapy, there are times when therapists need to initiate termination to uphold ethical obligations. At these times considerations of beneficence and/or nonmaleficence may override the client's autonomy. In fact, ethics codes discuss the need to terminate treatment if therapy is not helping or might be harmful, even when clients might express a desire to stay in therapy (more on this situation later). The obligation is to terminate a treatment that is not working and refer clients to sources of help that may be more effective. One possible acculturation stress occurs when our personal feelings of care and helpfulness come into conflict with our professional judgment that we cannot provide what some clients need.

Therapist-initiated Termination that's Too Soon or Too Late

In contrast to the situation above, some therapists, with some clients, with some problems, may seek to terminate therapy too soon or too late. Why do you think this might be the case? Speculate a bit about why therapists might be too soon or too late to terminate a therapy relationship. As you do, we invite you to reflect back on your journal entry from earlier in this chapter. Based on what you wrote, consider reasons why *you* may terminate soon or too late. If you think you will be making (or do make) perfect choices with all the clients you see – think again …

One reason therapists may initiate nonoptimal terminations might be predilections based on theoretical orientation. For example, at one end of the continuum are therapeutic approaches that encourage a thorough understanding of clients' personalities and comprehensive changes in many areas of client functioning. Therapists on this end of the continuum may be a little too hesitant to end therapy. On the other end of the continuum are therapy approaches that work on very specific problems. When the specific fear is reduced, for example, therapy is over. If clients have other issues, they can sign up for another course of treatment with the current therapist or another therapist.

Differences in judgment about when to terminate based on therapeutic orientation may reflect legitimate differences in approach. When clients have been well informed, it is not unethical to have therapy be somewhat longer or shorter than it would have been with another therapist. However, when these theoretical predilections become biases and override other concerns and values, therapists may be at risk of violating competence, beneficence, and other Ethical Foundations.

Another reason therapists may not terminate at an optimal time is differences in ethical reasoning – achieving the difficult balance that must be achieved between when actualizing the principles of autonomy and beneficence. Some therapists may give autonomy a little more weight and allow clients to make decisions about termination that are not the best. Here, clients may have derived more benefit from a little closer guidance from the therapist. Other therapists, perhaps using an assimilation strategy, might feel that their judgment of when to terminate – because it's so well informed by expertise – should be forcefully presented and accepted without concern. Once again, reasonable people can hold different ethical theories. We believe, of course, that these theories are most useful when they are applied in the context of virtues such as humility.

Another reason therapists may not end therapy at an optimal time is their own feelings, including their sense of completion, achievement, and helpfulness. Some people like small achievements in incremental stages. Other people like to look at achievements on a grander scale. Think of it this way: Some writers write limericks and celebrate the completion of each one, others write short stories, and still others do not feel like writers until they complete an epic novel.

As you look back on your journal entry, see if you can become more aware of your own tendencies to say "goodbye" either too soon or too late. These tendencies could reflect personal issues, such as commitment or the need to be a helper; personal feelings like guilt or achievement; or tendencies based on ethically relevant dimensions. Also, we invite you to think back to your own ethics autobiography and the values exercises you completed in chapter 1. How do you see your role as a therapist? Are you a lifelong guide? Or maybe a short-term consultant? What do you believe clients and you should get out of a successful therapy process? How might the answers to these questions influence your thoughts about termination?

Too Soon   Stopping treatment too soon might be considered *abandonment*, which several professional ethics codes specifically prohibit.

For example, the ACA Code (2005, A.11.a.) states: "Counselors do not abandon or neglect clients in counseling. Counselors assist in making appropriate arrangements for the continuation of treatment, when necessary, during interruptions such as vacations, illness, and following termination."

Sometimes stopping therapy too soon is stimulated or influenced by external factors: the insurance money runs out, one party is moving, or the therapist is retiring or changing positions. But sometimes there are internal reasons – the therapist may have some unresolved counter-transference, such as feelings of anger, boredom, or disgust. These feelings, of course, are a good indication that some consultation is necessary.

Too Late   The upper right box of Figure 9.1 represents cases in which therapists initiate termination too late. Perhaps they make a technical mistake and don't realize either that the client's needs have been met or will not be met by the current therapy. Thus, the therapist wants to continue therapy longer than is wise. Therapists may even convince clients who want to terminate that they should "hang in there." Why might therapists do this? The answers would include reasons for any unethical behavior, including incompetence, external pressures such as the financial benefit they get from clients, internal issues like the need to be needed and a lack of prudence or humility, or the combination of internal and external pressures involved in conflicts of interest.

Red Flag: *Sideline Solicitations*

Jenna has really appreciated the time her therapist, Dr Pak, has taken to explain lots of different things she could do to improve her condition. They've talked about hiking, nutrition, yoga, some more hiking, taking classes at the local community college, a little bit more about hiking, tai chi, and – you guessed it – hiking. One day while waiting to see Dr Pak, Jenna notices a new table in the waiting room. On it is a cardboard display with several copies of a book, *Hiking Trails in the Tri-State Area*. Jenna has to squint to see it, but she's stunned as she notices the author's name: Dr F. Pak. Alongside the books are several types of energy bars. She picks one up and reads part of the label: "Pack some energy for your hike with Pak's Energy Packs!"

Now Jenna feels a little strange. She can't help but wonder whether the hiking recommendation came from good professional judgment or was just a setup. She puts the bar down on the table and finds the energy to hike out of Dr Pak's office and over to the state board …

As you consider this case, don't be fooled into thinking that Dr Pak's behavior is so extreme that it couldn't apply to you. What if Dr Pak were not selling hiking materials but therapy materials – say, a very good self-help book? Should Dr Pak require the client to buy it? What if Dr Pak was the author of the book and stood to make a profit?

Journal Entry: *Better Never than Late*

Here is a story we heard from a friend in which the therapist's approach really created some bad feelings that were quite unnecessary:

> My therapist didn't seem to want to stop. She said she had a formula, that for every month I was in therapy we needed to spend a month in the termination process. I really got a lot out of the therapy, but I didn't see the need to spend that much time saying goodbye. So I just told her that we were finished. I've come to a reasonably good spot, and I'm ready to finish. For the next few weeks, I would get brief phone calls from her saying that she was still able to meet with me. I felt like she was trying too hard to keep me as a client. And it's a shame, because even though I enjoyed the work we did, I don't think I'll go back to her when I want therapy again.

In your journal, contemplate this story in terms of the concepts we've explored in this book. What is wrong with this picture? What values, motives, virtues, and acculturation strategies might the therapist be using? If you were a member of an ethics committee and received a complaint about this therapist's activities, would you judge that ethical principles were violated (which Foundations?), or was this more like an error in judgment that did not rise to the level of an ethical violation? What is the basis for your judgment?

Client-initiated Termination

In some therapeutic approaches, such as client-centered therapy, it is the client who generally makes the decision about termination. Ideally, the client will feel autonomous, safe, and healthy enough to suggest that therapy stop. You may think that the reaction of therapists to their clients' suggestions to stop treatment would be uniformly positive, especially when the therapy is ending with a positive outcome.

The reality, of course, is more complex. Along with feelings of happiness and fulfillment come feelings that can include sadness, rejection, resentment, and loss. Again, it is important for you to know some of your typical reactions to ending relationships. Of course, the negative feelings might be much more prominent when clients suggest ending therapy because therapy is not working for them. This kind of suggestion may challenge the irrational belief that many therapists hold that they are good people who can help anybody (Deutsch, 1984).

It's hard to stare failure in the face! It's hard to give up and refer your client to other therapists under any circumstances. But when a client suggests termination you may feel doubly bad because therapy failed, and you weren't on top of the situation enough to know exactly how bad it was! You may feel incompetent. You may feel jilted!

When referring a client to another therapist, O'Reilly (1987) suggests that therapists may experience the "transfer syndrome," which involves feelings of guilt, depression, and even relief. These feelings can be compounded by "fears of evaluation by peers or supervisors, anxiety concerning what the client might expose about him or her, and anxiety about the new placement" (Rice & Follette, 2003, p. 162). Thus, pretermination counseling sessions may be as important to therapists as they are to clients because they are opportunities for therapists to channel their anxiety into productive behaviors and reorient their values.

When therapy fails, it is especially important for you to be aware of these emotional reactions and think about your values, virtues, and principles. How much do you value being seen as omniscient vs. being seen as facilitating client growth? Part of respecting client autonomy is respecting their judgments and choices even though they make you feel bad. These are times when your virtues of compassion and humility have to be finely tuned. If you keep the value of client welfare uppermost in your mind, you may be better able to weather the emotional storms involved in termination. Remember that handling the termination well – making excellent referrals, doing excellent pretermination counseling – can create or maintain feelings of competence even in a failed therapy. These actions thus become good integration strategies.

Too Soon   Picture this: You are working with a client and thinking that you are just starting to make some progress. The client comes in and wants to terminate; she says that everything is fine. Here, the client may be initiating termination too soon. How do you handle this situation? How do you balance your judgment about what is in the client's best interests with their right to terminate?

To deal with this situation, you need to think about some informed consent issues. For example, you need to think through how much information you provide, what options you discuss, and how much you encourage the client to continue. Sometimes this is a relatively easy matter because you have objective evidence – from a competent and careful assessment – that the client's own goals have not been met. At other times the discussion may be more of a true negotiation about goals between equal partners.

Here's a variation on the theme of the client needing more treatment: Imagine a situation in which your client's initial goals have been met and the client suggests termination. You believe, however, that the client could benefit from additional treatment. For example, the initial depression has lifted, but the client could still benefit from some assertiveness training that you are competent to provide. The decision to suggest continued therapy, when clearly the client's initial goals have been met, is a tricky one. You want to respect clients' desires, but you also want to provide information with which clients can make better decisions. The decision about how much information to provide at this point mirrors our discussion of how much information to provide at the beginning of treatment.

Food for Thought: *How to Suggest More Treatment*

You are seeing a client who has been very successful in dealing with the issues he came in with. However, you have strong feelings that some issues of the client that the two of you didn't deal with in therapy are likely to cause trouble in the foreseeable future. Which of the following statements are you most likely to make? What acculturation strategies might the statement represent? Might there be situations in which you are more likely to make one of the other statements?

- It is my professional opinion that you need more treatment to deal with a few other issues that have arisen in the course of our work together. I would be the best person to continue to help you.
- I understand your desire to terminate. I agree that this is a great place to stop. As we do, let me share with you some impressions I have about some things that you might want to work on later if you decide to come back or if you decide to work with somebody else.
- I'm glad we've completed our contract. I wish you continued success in the future. If you decide to come back, feel free to contact me.
- You really can't go yet. Please come back next week.

How do you know when to suggest that your client add some goals and continue therapy? Here are some possible indicators that your suggestion to continue treatment is a good one and well done:

- The invitation to continue should not come as a surprise to your client. In fact, if the therapy has been good you might have been talking with your client all along about various directions the therapy could take.

- You should be able to offer the idea as a low-pressure suggestion, not a fiat. If you find that you really *need* the client to accept your invitation, it may be time for some consultation.
- The explanation for why the client should continue should make perfect sense – it should feel like an organic outgrowth of the work you have been doing.

Too Late   For some therapists, the most difficult box in Figure 9.1 is the lower right – when therapists judge that the therapy is over (either successfully or unsuccessfully) but the client feels like therapy should go on. This may indicate client *dependency*. Clients may start talking about new goals for therapy that don't seem like they are amenable to treatment or workable for you. Or, the client may say, "You know, I think I'd like to work on my relationship with my 22nd cousin Sadie. That should take another year." Another indication of dependency is when the client simply cannot come up with any reasons to continue but is adamant about not wanting to stop.

We have talked about ways of preventing dependency, such as having a good informed consent process that includes a discussion of termination and being specific about goals. But when it happens, the contrast between the principles of autonomy and beneficence is very stark, and the feelings and reactions we've been discussing may be especially salient. Here's the acculturation stress: Personally we may feel like we can see clients as long as they want, but, from a professional standpoint, we have the obligation to terminate therapy because it is best for the client.

Green Flags: *Good Goals and Ethical Endings*

Having good goals right from the beginning makes the end of therapy easier. Consider this:

Karyn has been working with Dr Brooks for several months. They have been using a behavioral approach to decrease Karyn's anxiety in social situations. Karyn enjoys most of her consulting work activities, but the networking and sales were really troubling her for a long time until her therapy with Dr Brooks.

For the past several sessions, Karyn has been talking about how delighted she is with her progress, and how everything seems to be going well. She has been able to go to parties and "schmooze" quite well. Dr Brooks says, "Well, you know, Karyn, we've talked several times recently about it being close to the end of therapy. Maybe we ought to call the next session our last one, given that you've done what you've set out to do."

Karyn replies, "Oh. But I really like coming here. It just feels so good to be here."

Dr Brooks replies evenly, "It's really been a pleasure to work with you. And throughout our work, we've discussed your goals and now it seems you've met all of them. Can you think of other therapeutic goals you'd like to achieve?"

Karyn grimaces, as if she's just tasted a lemon. She knows Dr Brooks is very straightforward, and she's finding it difficult to be confronted about ending therapy. At the same time, she knows this has been coming for a while. She even feels a little relieved that Dr Brooks is not letting her get away with coming to therapy just because it's become a habit. "Well, when you put it that way, I guess we really are finished with our work. I just find it hard to say goodbye."

"Yes, let's consider that during our last session next week. What I hear you saying is that you agree that your goals have been met –"

"Oh, yes, definitely," Karyn says.

"But you're also saying that it's hard to leave, it's hard to say goodbye."

They spend the last few minutes of that session recapping the gains that Karyn has made. At the next session, they say their goodbyes. Dr Brooks offers to see Karyn again when there is something to deal with. Karyn feels really good – not only that her therapist helped her with her social skills and her anxiety, but because her therapist was upfront with her about the purpose of therapy. She knows that, if problems develop in the future, there's somebody there for her.

In sum, all these decisions have clearly to do with clinical decisions and issues. They also have to do with your own values about what good you can provide on what level. You can provide good by doing good therapy and by allowing clients to end therapy and try out some freedom, initiative, and self-determination. You can actualize your value of doing good for clients by a prudent referral with humility and compassion.

Worst Termination Ever: Getting Complained Against

The worst case scenario for most of us is when clients not only inform us of their desire to terminate, but also tell us that they are filing a complaint against us with the state board or ethics committee. It is beyond the scope of this book to provide detailed suggestions for how to handle complaints against you and your practice (see Chauvin & Remley, 1996; Thomas, 2005). For now, although we hope you will never face this situation, we also want to acknowledge the possibility. It is hard to think of a more acute acculturation crisis (Berry & Kim, 1988) and this situation strikes at the heart of our values of helping and our carefully honed professional virtues. You want to be prepared for the possibility.

Some therapists may choose a separation strategy – they may discount the ethical standards they are accused of violating. Thomas wrote, "If they recognize the violation but disagree with the rule, they may believe their actions were justified and, therefore, may feel indignant and incredulous" (2005, p. 427). In our service on ethics committees, we have also seen all too often that therapists will counterattack or pathologize clients who make complaints. We have also heard about what might be extreme assimilation responses – therapists simply turn in their licenses rather than undergo an investigation of the complaint.

But there is a third response. Therapists who have been complained against still have the opportunity to take a positive approach. If we are complained against, we can take the complaint seriously and use our reasoning and choice-making skills in our response. "The ability to articulate to the board a clear understanding of mistakes and related ethical issues and to demonstrate a commitment to rectifying problems are [*sic*] likely to result in improved practices and to augment the [psychotherapist's] defense" (Thomas, 2005, p. 431).

Thomas goes on to say that the complaint process can give us an opportunity to learn. "Being the subject of a complaint may provide the impetus for initiating ... changes. Time and money spent on required supervision or education may feel more worthwhile to [psychotherapists] who take an active role in determining how the experience can further their professional goals" (2005, p. 432).

At such stressful times, a positive approach includes taking time to care for ourselves – taking some time off, getting some personal support, etc. It also includes stepping back and perhaps re-acculturating. We may need to meditate about our fundamental motivations and values – what we wrote on our graduate school applications or our ethics autobiographies.

Part III
The Ethical Ceiling

10

Putting It All Together
Toward Ethical Excellence

"How do you get to Carnegie Hall? Practice, practice, practice."
Old joke, attributed to Henry Youngman

We have our treadmill (see chapter 1), we have read all the directions, and we are familiar with all the programs of which the machine is capable. But are we in shape? If someone asks us if we are comfortable with "Fat Burn Program #4," can we say "yes" merely because we know what page it's on and perhaps because we tried the first few minutes of it once? Of course not. Knowledge *of* the machine is only part of our ability to work *on* the machine. Similarly, our knowledge *of* ethics is only part of our ability to *be* ethically excellent.

By now, you know that there is no magic formula for considering ethical issues. But you have tried out some of the "programs" via journal entries, food for thought exercises, and stories of green and red flags. You have discovered some acculturation strategies that you use more than others. If you've followed us and accepted our invitations in the first nine chapters, you may be experiencing two conflicting feelings. First, you may be feeling some sense of accomplishment. And rightly so! Second, you also may be feeling unsure that you "know all the rules" or can react ethically in all the situations you (will) face as a psychotherapist. In other words, you may feel that your professional ethical identity is not totally formed. As we've mentioned before, your ethical identity, your acculturation into the profession, will be an ongoing, lifelong process.

Your next task in this process is to practice and refine the skills we have introduced you to. In this chapter we will help you review some of what you have learned in the form of cases you can work through. We will also help you look ahead to the next steps in your ethical identity development.

Practice, Practice, Practice

In this section we invite you to revisit all that we've done and to prac-tice with some short cases. You can tackle these cases in several differ-ent ways. You can use the choice-making process that we covered in chapter 3. You can list the values, virtues, and motivations that you would, could, or should bring to bear. You can formulate alternative courses of action and decide which ones are most ethically excellent – which ones represent integration and which ones represent the other acculturation strategies. You can write down your gut feelings and your first impressions of a course of action and then test your gut against the Ethical Foundations. However you choose to undertake each case, we encourage you to try different approaches, to continue looking at the intersection of personal and professional ethics, and to practice the kinds of reasoning and other skills that you are *least* comfortable with at the moment. This is not a test! Feel free to go back and review por-tions of the book as you consider each case.

The Case of the Disrespected Doctor

Dr Gillespie has been seeing John for several weeks. Over the last couple sessions she has noticed that John has been speaking in more and more disrespectful ways. He makes disparaging comments about many groups of people, some of which represent her upbringing, her sexual preference, her political views, and just about everything else. Dr Gillespie doesn't know whether John is expressing these views to attack her or not – in fact, she's not even sure John knows her sexual orientation or political views. But one day, he talks about "stupid therapists," and then says, "If the shoe fits!"

Dr Gillespie knows that the ethical principle of justice says that John is just as entitled to therapy as any other person. Indeed, he does seem to be doing some therapeutic work – some of which is related to his disrespectful speech but most of which is not related at all to the things he says about her and her values. She also knows that one of her most prized virtues is compassion and respect for all people. But she's human, and she's angry.

Dr Gillespie comes to you for a consultation. How do you help her? Among the questions to consider:

- What values, virtues, and motivations may Dr Gillespie have, and how might they conflict with each other?
- What alternative courses of action might Dr Gillespie have, and what acculturation strategies might they represent?
- What values, virtues, and motivations might govern *your* approach to consultation with Dr Gillespie?
- What alternatives do *you* have, and what acculturation strategies do they represent?

The Case of the Indispensable Insurance

You are seeing a client for some marital problems. He's a little sad, a little anxious, but doesn't really come close to fitting any psychiatric diagnosis that insurance will cover. He does not have enough money to be able to afford therapy without insurance and his insurance will not pay for therapy without a diagnosis. Some of the following thoughts run through your head: "Giving a diagnosis is just a formality. This is really what insurance is for. Anyway, my treatment will save the insurance company money in the long run by preventing my client from having a full-blown depression. Besides, insurance companies are so big that they won't miss a little of their money."

- What might be the arguments on both sides of the issue of providing a diagnosis for insurance coverage?
- If you were the client how would you see the issue?
- What about "gray area" situations – for example, what if the client was one symptom shy of a reimbursable diagnosis?

Here's a variation of the story: You are doing marital therapy for the client and his wife, but the insurance only covers individual therapy.

- How would you report your work to the insurance company?
- Would it be ethical or not to report that you were doing "individual therapy" for the husband with the wife as a "collateral contact?"

Our view is that intentionally assigning a diagnosis that is not accurate is unethical. To get paid by an insurance company for intentionally assigning inaccurate diagnosis is called insurance fraud.

Such a behavior might be evidence of a separation strategy, and maybe even marginalization.

The Case of the Very Variable Values

You are seeing a client who is very underprivileged, in her 40s, living on public assistance, and who has struggled with depression for most of her life. Your goal in the therapy is to provide some much-needed support and help her develop a few more life skills. In her conversation one day she talks about her brother. You are happy to hear that she is much happier now that her brother has moved back to the state following the death of both their parents. In fact, he has moved in with her.

As her story unfolds, you learn that the brother is the source of great comfort to your client. She says they spend most nights together watching television – this is all she can really afford and she has always had difficulty making friends. Your client tells you that sometimes they hold each other as they watch a particularly sad movie on TV.

One day your client tells you that she and her brother have had sexual relations. She says it's OK because she's had a hysterectomy and can't become pregnant.

What is your *personal* reaction? What does your gut tell you to do? What personal values are at stake? If you weren't her therapist, how would you respond to this information? Why? What would you do if a relative – say, a cousin – told you this? Think of one of your good friends; what if they told you this?

What is your *professional* reaction? What are your therapeutic obligations? What values drive your deliberations?

What if the client weren't "underprivileged"? What if she were able to bear children? What if she were a favorite client of yours? What if she were wealthy? What if she were from a different ethnic background than you?

The Case of the Tempting Tickets

You are a psychotherapist in private practice. Pat, your first client of the day, is very attractive to you and one of your favorites. Pat offers you some extra tickets to an event you really want to attend but couldn't get tickets to. Your client got them for free. How do you respond to Pat's offer? Why? How would you justify your response?

As you think about this scenario, be aware of how you read the story. How did you interpret the word "favorite?" Did you assume that Pat was offering to go with you to the event? Was Pat male or female? When we said that Pat was "attractive," how did you picture that attraction? Sexual? Romantic? Emotional? Intellectual? Financial?

Now, reflect on this: What would need to be different in this scenario for your response to Pat to be different? What if, for example, you already had tickets? Or what if you didn't want tickets? What if Pat were very wealthy? What if Pat were your *least* favorite client? Think about some other variations and how they might influence your thinking.

To broaden the discussion, think about these questions:

- What kinds of people in your life do you find it hard to say "no" to? Why?
- What are your usual strategies for trying to refuse a request from these folks?
- How might the elements of the culture of psychotherapy make it easier or harder to refuse a request?

For this case, we wanted to share the following story:

Green Flags: *Beneficial Boundary Bolstering, Effective Ethical Explanations, and Ethical Explorations*

One day, Benny, a psychotherapist himself, invites his therapist, Dr Stan Tall, to a football game. Benny was given these tickets for free and feels that he can tolerate some small boundary crossings. He's not really bribing his therapist nor even trying to butter him up. However, Dr Tall refuses the tempting offer: "I really appreciate your invitation, but my policy is not to accept social invitations from clients. I really respect you and I respect the therapy we've been working so hard at. To keep the therapy working well, we need to keep it 'pure' and not add other types of interactions to it." Benny is taken aback for a moment, feeling as if Dr Tall is not respecting him. However, before he can react Dr Tall continues, "I'm wondering what it felt like to ask me to the football game, and to have me refuse." Now, Benny sees that Dr Tall was not showing disrespect for him, but showing respect for the process of therapy. He knows that it's going to be an uncomfortable session in which he has to think carefully about his motivations. But he is surprisingly relieved to know that Dr Tall is so consistent in his approach.

GREEN

The Case of the Complicated and Complicating Complaint

You have been seeing a 6-year-old boy for about a year. The parents have been in a nasty divorce, which is what prompted therapy. The mother says she has legal custody of the son and doesn't want you to work with the father. The father, after seeing you a couple times, refuses to come in and appears to be hostile to any form of therapy for himself. In fact, he has asked you to terminate treatment with his son – a request you refused because (a) the mother signed the consent form and (b) you feel that the child is benefiting from the therapy.

One day you get a letter indicating that the father is filing a formal complaint against you with the ethics committee of your professional association. The complaint says that you have sided with the mother against the father and that you have acted incompetently. Your attorney tells you that the complaint appears to be without merit and will probably be dismissed. But there is always the possibility that he will file a complaint with the state board.

You see the son twice a month for therapy and have a good working relationship with him. At the same time, you are feeling very frustrated with the parents and their manipulation of you. You feel resentment toward the father and all the inconvenience he is causing in your practice, not to mention the assault on your professional integrity. On top of all of this you are nervous about the possible outcomes of his complaints. The question: Do you terminate therapy with the child or continue to see him?

What is your initial response? How might your values and your ethical culture(s) of origin be influencing your judgment? What Ethical

Foundations are relevant to this case and how do they relate to each other? What courses of action might there be and which one seems best? Why? What arguments can be made for the other courses of action? What facts of the case would have to change for you to change your course of action?

Put yourself in the role of the child, the mother, and the father. For example, ask yourself, "What if I were a 6 year old and my parents were divorcing and my therapist said to me, 'We have to discontinue treatment …'"?

Now, put yourself in the position of an ethics committee member. What if you were on a committee that heard a case …

1. brought by the mother after the therapist terminated therapy with the child, OR
2. brought by the father after the therapist refused to accede to his request that therapy be terminated with his son, OR
3. brought by an advocate for the child, for *either* terminating or not terminating.

The Case of the Relative Referral

You are a very well-trained and competent family therapist in a small city. You have been seeing a couple off and on over a period of five years. They came to you when their marriage hit a rough spot. Your typical approach is solution focused and thus far this approach has been very effective with the couple. Based on your ongoing assessment, the relationship seems to be getting stronger.

One day the husband calls you and asks for a referral for himself. He would like to go into individual therapy with somebody who uses the same approach you do. He says, "I'd come to see you because I really like how you work, but I know that I can't because I'm already seeing you as part of a couple."

"That's right," you answer, sure of your ethical ground. "That would be a conflict of interest for me and a multiple relationship for us. But I'll think about some possible referrals and give you a couple of names of people I trust."

The next day you call the client with the names of the best two therapists in town who use the same approach you do. "The first person is Samuel Howard, an excellent therapist."

"I know him!" your client says. "He's a tennis buddy of mine!"

"Well, that leaves him out, obviously." You share your other name – someone your client is not familiar with. You're just about to end the call on that successful note when your client says, "I'd really like one or two more names, just in case I don't get along with this person. I'd feel much more comfortable with a choice of folks."

"Let me think about it and get back to you." You already know that there are very few people in town who use your approach. The good news is that there is one more person you know who is a good therapist – well-trained, seasoned, very ethical, and able to be very successful with your client. The bad news is: this person is your spouse/partner!

Here are some of your alternative courses of action:

- You could tell your client you don't have any other referrals to offer.
- You could give the client your spouse's name as a referral and not tell the client you are related to the person (you have different last names). After all, you and your spouse never talk about the details of cases you are seeing, including identities, so there is little if any danger of either of you finding out things you shouldn't know.
- You could give the client the referral and explain to him that the therapist is your spouse. You could explain your policy as a professional couple about not sharing names or details about clients, and offer to answer any questions the client has.
- You could discuss with your client the possibility of working with someone who has a different approach and that this would probably yield a larger list of referrals.

What other options might there be? Of the options listed, which one appears to be the *most* ethical course of action? Which option appears to be the *least* ethical? What are the pros and cons for each option? Which options would represent – for you – integration, assimilation, and separation strategies? Why?

What if the referral was for a family member whom you were not seeing – a father, mother, sibling, son, or daughter? How would that change the issues and considerations? What other facts of the case would alter the choices you make?

The Case of Previous Contact

Our last two cases in this section incorporate flag stories. This story represents the green flags of Beneficial Boundary Bolstering, Effective Ethical Explanations, and Ethical Explorations (see chapter 4):

> My wife and I went to a psychotherapist for marital counseling. We all sat down in her office. We were surprised when the first thing she said was, "I think I know you." It only took a few minutes for her to remember that we'd played charades together at the home of a mutual acquaintance. I didn't really remember that one incident, but I was impressed that she brought it up and encouraged us to think about whether that would get in the way. We decided that the one contact wasn't enough to skew our impressions of each other, and, anyway, we had pretty much lost touch with those acquaintances. But it felt good to know that our therapist was really attuned to the ethical stuff and to the potential problems that might develop. She wound up being a great therapist for us. The funny thing is, a year or so after we stopped therapy, we wound up at a party at our mutual acquaintance's house! My wife and I felt really comfortable saying hello, as people do at parties. The therapist smiled and said hello. Of course, we didn't go out of our way to socialize with her, and she didn't initiate more contact either.

Think about variations of this story that may not have turned out so well. What would those be? What changes in the therapist's behavior, values, virtues, acculturation strategy, etc. might you identify in less excellent versions? What would you have done if you were in the therapist's position? Why? What if you were in the clients' position and the therapist said she wouldn't see you?

The Case of the Controversial Comment

This story represents the red flag of Intimations of Inappropriate Intimacy:

> "You look good," Dr Tall said to Ms Reeves as she entered the office.
> "What?" she asked. "Why did you say that?" This was unusual behavior for Dr Tall.

"Well, I remembered that you were going for your job interview today, and we've been working on your assertiveness skills in preparation. You look very professional."

Ms Reeves felt a bit relieved at this explanation. She remembered her previous therapist, Dr Kidder, who used to make comments about her appearance all the time. She felt a bit flattered at first, but then she had felt uncomfortable as Dr Kidder's comments on how nice she looked became more frequent. Then he started asking her personal questions about her social and family life. These questions didn't feel right – somehow, they seemed like prying rather than therapy.

Ms Reeves decided not to fire Dr Tall for this one remark, because it was not a very strong red flag. It could certainly have been an innocent comment, and he'd never done anything else to suggest to Ms Reeves that he was trying to blur any boundaries or get too intimate with her. "So," she says to herself, "I'll just file this away for possible future reference. Anyway, I want to talk about this job interview!"

What is your initial response to Dr Tall's actions and why? What is your initial response to Ms Reeve's thoughts and reactions? If you were Dr Tall's supervisor and heard about this exchange, what, if anything, would you say to him and why?

Journal Entry: *Goals of Psychotherapy*

It is easy to say that therapists are ethically obligated to help clients reach their goals. That's part of the culture of psychotherapy. But what if clients' goals are or seem inappropriate? Do those goals still get the same priority? One way to begin answering these questions is to explore both appropriate and inappropriate therapeutic goals.

Some client goals are clearly within the province of therapy: fewer arguments with a partner, alleviation of symptoms of depression or anxiety, becoming better able to deal with authority figures. Other goals that clients may have are clearly inappropriate or irrelevant to psychotherapy: sexual activity with the therapist, financial security, plugging up that leak in the downstairs bathroom. Some goals, however, constitute a gray area.

Part 1 To begin the exercise, make a list of goals that clients might have in their lives and might present to the therapist as work for therapy.

Part 2 Consider the conditions under which each would be a legitimate therapeutic goal. For example, would it be appropriate for a person to come to therapy to:

- get the unconditional support they don't get at home?
- develop a business that pollutes the environment, cheats the government, or exploits customers?
- feel more comfortable about their submissiveness to their partner?
- decide to end their life because of a terminal illness?

Part 3 List some goals that therapists might have for clients. These goals might be appropriate, inappropriate, or in a gray area. Indicate which category you think each goal on your list falls under. Here are some examples we have thought of: Therapists might have a goal to:

- make clients better able to make decisions in and about therapy itself;
- make clients better consumers of psychotherapy.

Or therapists might be focused on helping their clients:

- be more assertive;
- use more of their potential;
- give up some of their religious beliefs that the therapist sees as irrational;
- become more comfortable with their sexuality;
- accept the constraints other people place on them because of their disability, or religion, or ethnic identification, or sexual orientation, or some other characteristic;
- see them (the therapists) as potential romantic partners.

Part 4   Look back over your lists of goals and see which goals might cause the most disagreement between therapists and clients. That is, which goals might clients have for themselves that therapists would not consider appropriate or relevant? Which goals might therapists have for clients that clients might not like or might consider inappropriate?

Part 5   Let us explore the issue of implicit vs. explicit goals. Take a few of the goals you identified in Part 3 – the ones that therapists might have for clients. Put yourself in the place of a therapist who has the best interests of the client at heart. Which goals would you share with the client and which ones would you keep to yourself? Then, put yourself in the place of the client and ask yourself which goals your therapist might have for you that you would want to know about.

Ethics Policies

Picture this: You have a portable flash drive on which you keep your client records. This is very convenient because you can work on reports and billing both at home and at the office. But where do you keep the drive when you are not working? In your brief case? A drawer in your desk? A locked file cabinet?

You might not think that such a mundane question would arise in an ethics book. But imagine this: You lose your drive, or it is stolen. (It is much easier to lose a small flash drive than an entire computer.) You casually mention this to a client of yours who promptly files an ethics complaint against you because you have compromised her confidentiality.

Many aspects of our practice may not seem directly related to abstract ethical principles or even specific professional standards. But virtually all of our behaviors have ethics components and are reflections of our professional identity. Thus, it's useful to think in advance about the types of everyday decisions we are or will be making, and to formulate policies – preexisting rules or guidelines – that are consistent with, or actualize, our highest professional principles, virtues, and values.

In Appendix B we've listed many (but maybe not all!) the areas about which you could have policies. As you think about these policies, it is a good idea to make explicit the ethical justifications for your approach.

Let's look a little closer at a couple of the policies in Appendix B. Look at Policies #3 and #4. How do you know when you are competent? Think of a client you are very competent to see. How did you determine that you were competent? Would an ethics committee agree? What and how much would have to change about this client before you would consider yourself not competent? More severe symptoms? Different ethnic background? Different gender? Older, younger?

Take a look at Policy #10 regarding coverage for evenings, weekends, and vacation times. What do you say on your phone message for clients who are experiencing a crisis, or for other reasons want to talk to you outside of their regular office appointments? Is it enough to be available only during regular business hours? Where do you tell clients to go – whom do you tell them to talk to – when you are not available?

Journal Entry: Cultures

Go back to the journal entry you completed in chapter 4: "My Current Location on the Road to Multicultural Competence." Notice the three cultures you feel you know a lot about and the three you know little or nothing about. Now, go back through the book and find several exercises that didn't have any specific reference to culture. Make the people in those exercises members of each of the cultures you know a lot about. How does that change things? Do this exercise again and make the people in the exercises a member of the cultures you know little or nothing about. What changes? What steps might you take to improve your multicultural competence?

Ethics Autobiography – Update

As your final task for this book, it's time to revisit and perhaps revise your ethics autobiography. In preparation, reflect upon the writing and exercises you did as you've proceeded through this book: What exercises did you like doing? What kinds of activities did you resist? For example, you may notice that you loved the motivations part, but not the virtues. You never really "got" how separation works or why it's not the most effective acculturation strategy.

Journal Entry: *Ethics Autobiography Update*

Reread the autobiography parts 1 and 2 that you completed in chapters 1 and 4. Now you can work on a revision that will serve you for the next phase of your training or career. What parts of the autobiography do you need to change? Are there thoughts you'd like to add? How might you increase your use of integration strategies? Where do you need work on virtues, values, and social awareness? In addition, how would you build in answers to the following questions?

- What behaviors do I give up (with some individuals) by being a professional (e.g., dating, sex, gossip, self-disclosure)?
- What do I *gain* by being a professional (e.g., watching people grow, appropriate use of knowledge and skill, gratitude, money)?

Add one more section to the autobiography: Make a list of your strengths, those aspects of ethical acculturation at which you find yourself articulate and confident. Then, make a list of the other aspects – those for which the words, feelings, and thoughts do not come so quickly. There is your list of what you can do to facilitate your development as a professional.

Toward Ethical Excellence

Here are several final points we want to share with you before you close the book. First, this book is ending, but your professional journey toward ethical excellence is not. Second, you have not been on an "ethical treadmill" to win a race but to increase your ethical endurance and stamina. Third, you do not "win" ethics by following the rules or by avoiding complaints but you can become more ethically excellent as you work toward understanding yourself and the culture of psychotherapy. In positive ethics there is no endpoint because we continue to change, to gain insight, and to improve our virtues, behaviors, and acculturation strategies. Striving for excellence is a process that keeps us going as professionals. Thus, you are on the treadmill to achieve, and continue to achieve, your personal – and professional – best.

We encourage you to look back at this book and at your ethics autobiography and journal entries on a regular basis – not just when you are in some ethical difficulty. We bet that each time you look back at what you've done you'll find something new and useful.

A Final Word

The relationship between authors and readers is yet another type of professional relationship with its own set of expectations, role obligations, and boundaries. We hope we have fulfilled our obligation to provide you with an experience that has enhanced your development and allowed you to fulfill your own obligations – to yourself and to the profession. We wish you much success and our last invitation to you is to share your reactions and experiences with this book with us. Here are our email addresses:

Sharon: sharon.anderson@colostate.edu
Mitch: mitchell.handelsman@ucdenver.edu

Appendix A

Possible Information to Be Shared with Clients

Much of this information is from Pomerantz & Handelsman, 2004 and Handelsman and Galvin, 1988.

Issues to Address about the Logistics of Therapy

- How often you'll meet for therapy
- The length or time of each session
- How appointment times are scheduled (phone, email, answering service, etc.)
- Your usual availability during the week
- How appointments can be changed when necessary
- How to reach you in case of an emergency
- Your backup coverage when you aren't available
- Whether or not you are willing to do therapy over the phone or over the Internet
- Your fee structure and how you handle no-shows
- How you are set up to receive payments
- How you will handle the situation if the client falls behind in payments
- Your policy for raising fees
- If the client decides to use insurance:
    - how much and what kind of information you will be required to share with the insurance company (diagnosis, symptoms, and other information)
    - the impact the insurance company can have on the therapy
- The possible issues if the insurance company and you disagree about treatment

Issues to Address about the Therapeutic Process

- The therapeutic approach you propose based on the client's goals and concerns
- What the research says about your approach and the client's concerns
- Your therapeutic approach and how you understand change
- How your therapeutic approach is structured and whether or not you follow a preplanned format
- Any estimate you have about the length of therapy
- How the two of you will:
  1. measure therapeutic progress
  2. know when your work together is done
  3. know when therapy is not working and discuss what options are available to you and the client
- The benefits of your therapeutic approach
- The risks of your therapeutic approach
- Assessments or tests you might have the client complete
- The type of issues or concern that you don't feel competent to address
- Your connection(s) with prescribing physicians
- The percentage of your clients that improve and how you know this information
- The percentage of your clients that don't improve and even get worse and how you know this information
- The other types of therapy that work (according to research) with their concerns or goals
- The risks and benefits of no therapy for people with their type of concerns or goal

Issues to Address about Ethics Policies

- Professional organizations you belong to
- The codes of ethics you use or you are bound to (Be ready to hand a copy of your current ethical code to your client in case he or she asks for a copy.)
- Ethical guidelines you use regarding confidentiality

- The kind of records you keep and who has access to them (insurance companies, supervisors, employers, others)
- The conditions where you are required to breach confidentiality
- How you will handle confidentiality when it comes to family members
- How HIPPA regulations and other governmental regulations influence confidentiality of your records
- How you handle boundary issues or multiple relationships with clients
- Who the client can talk with if they have a complaint about therapy which can't be worked out between the two of you

Issues About You and Self-disclosure

- Your policy about therapist self-disclosure
- The kind(s) of degree you have and what they were in
- The institution(s) you received them from
- Your license as a psychotherapist
- The number of years you have been doing psychotherapy
- How long you have been helping people with the client's sort of problem(s)
- The entity that regulates your psychotherapy practice
- Other credentials that you have acquired that suggest you have additional training or have gained additional expertise
- If you are under supervision, who your supervisor is, and how the client can contact him or her
- Some of your basic values that guide your work and your life
- Whether you work from a religious framework (e.g., "Are we going to pray together? Are you going to assign Bible verses?")
- Political or moral issues that you feel strongly about
- Your views about _____? [Here, we invite you to fill in the blank with whatever issues you feel strongly about that you might feel compelled to address: Abortion; civil rights; homosexual marriage; home schooling; war; the new zoning ordinance downtown; parenting styles; gay rights; gun control; terrorism.]

Appendix B

Policy Areas

These are some of the areas in which you might want to have written policies. Some of these will be familiar, as we've talked about them in this book. Others will be new to you. Each policy should be formulated with consideration given to all the acculturation tasks we've covered, such as becoming aware of your values, virtues, motivations, ethical codes, and preferred acculturation strategies. You also will need to adapt your general policies depending on:

- the context of your practice (agency, group private practice, etc.);
- the range of your clients (diagnosis, SES, gender, religion, ethnic group, etc.);
- the types of clients you consider difficult.

Remember that this is not an exhaustive list of policy areas (although it is exhausting ...). But it will get you started, no?

1. How do I dress?
2. What objects (pictures, diplomas, awards, political material, etc.) do I display in my office?
3. How do I determine my competence to treat a client?
4. What kind of clients am I incompetent to treat?
5. Forms of address – what do I want to be called by clients?
6. What preappointment information do I send to clients?
7. Informed consent:
    a. What do I tell all clients?
    b. What are the risks of my therapy?
    c. How do I tell clients the information they need to know?
    d. How do I address client questions?

     e. How do I assess what information particular clients might need to know?

     f. How do I document consent? Refusal? Assent?

     g. Do I use contracts?

8. What rights do clients have?

     a. consent;

     b. termination;

     c. second opinion;

     d. asking questions;

     e. rights to records.

9. How do I formulate the goals of treatment?

10. Coverage for vacations, weekends, other absences?

11. Emergencies?

12. Extratherapy contacts:

     a. phone calls;

     b. collateral contacts.

13. Invitations from clients for extra-therapy contact (social events, life events).

     a. What are my criteria for accepting and rejecting invitations?

14. Confidentiality:

     a. releases of information;

     b. privilege and other legal issues;

     c. requests for information from others;

     d. how do I send records?

     e. what is my complete list of exceptions to confidentiality, including abuse reporting, court orders, and other legal requirements?

15. Records

     a. storage – computer, files, etc.;

     b. disposal;

     c. retention of records;

     d. deleting obsolete records;

     e. sharing records with clients, colleagues;

     f. plans for moving, retiring, death;

     g. what is the format of my records?

     h. what are the components of my records?

16. Accepting and giving gifts

17. Finances:

a. fees for sessions, other contacts, emergencies, phone calls, testimony, etc.;
b. raising fees;
c. negotiating fees for new clients, clients who change circumstances, etc.;
d. missed and cancelled appointments;
e. billing and collecting fees;
f. bartering.
18. Advertising and public statements
19. Safety issues
a. How do I deal with clients who seem to be getting angry?
b. How do I deal with suicidal gestures, threats, behaviors?
c. How do I deal with threats from clients, others?
20. Termination and referral
a. How do I inform clients about the conditions under which termination and/or referral take place?
b. How do I terminate?
c. How do I refer?
d. How do I conduct pretermination (prereferral) counseling?
21. Knowledge of unprofessional conduct by colleagues
a. How do I talk with colleagues about concerns I have about their behavior?
b. What is my threshold for reporting the unethical conduct of colleagues?
22. If you are sued or complained against to an ethics committee, who are you going to call?
1. attorney?
2. insurance carrier?
3. risk management office at your agency?
4. therapist?
5. family?
6. colleagues?
23. Touching

References

Abeles, N. (1980). Teaching ethical principles by means of values confrontations. *Psychotherapy: Theory, Research and Practice, 17,* 384–391.

Ahia, C. E., & Martin, D. (1993). The danger-to-self-or-others exception to confidentiality. In T. P. Remley (Ed.), ACA legal series (Vol. 9). Alexandria, VA: American Counseling Association.

American Association for Marriage and Family Therapy (2001). *Code of ethics.* Washington, DC: Author.

American Counseling Association. (2005). *Code of ethics.* Alexandria, VA: Author.

American Psychological Association. (2002). Ethical principles of psychologists and code of conduct. *American Psychologist, 51,* 1060–1073.

Anderson, S. K., & Kitchener, K. S. (1996). A critical incident study of non-romantic/nonsexual relationships between psychologists and former clients. *Professional Psychology: Research and Practice, 27,* 59–66.

Anderson, S. K., & Kitchener, K. S. (1998). Nonsexual post-therapy relationships: A conceptual framework to assess ethical risks. *Professional Psychology: Research and Practice, 29,* 91–99.

Anderson, S. K., & Middleton, V. A. (2005a). Introduction: An awakening to privilege, oppression, and discrimination. In S. K. Anderson & V. A. Middleton (Eds.), *Explorations in privilege, oppression and discrimination.* Belmont, CA: Thomson Brooks/Cole.

Anderson, S. K., & Middleton, V. A. (Eds.) (2005b). *Explorations in privilege, oppression and discrimination.* Belmont, CA: Thomson Brooks/Cole.

Anderson, S. K., Wagoner, H., & Moore, G. K. (2006). Ethical choice: An outcome of being, blending, and doing. In P. Williams & S. K. Anderson (Eds.), *Law and ethics in coaching: How to solve and avoid difficult problems in your practice* (pp. 39–61). Hoboken, NJ: John Wiley & Sons.

Appelbaum, P. S., Lidz, C. W., & Meisel, A. (1987). *Informed consent: Legal theory and clinical practice.* New York: Oxford University Press.

Baird, B. N. (1999). *The internship, practicum, and field placement handbook*. Upper Saddle River, NJ: Prentice Hall.

Barnett, J. E., Erickson Cornish, J. A., Goodyear, R. K., & Lichtenberg, J. W. (2007). Commentaries on the ethical and effective practice of clinical supervision. *Professional Psychology: Research and Practice, 38*, 268–275.

Barnett, J. E., Wise, E. H., Johnson-Greene, D., & Bucky, S. F. (2007). Informed consent: Too much of a good thing or not enough? *Professional Psychology: Research and Practice, 38*, 179–186.

Bashe, A., Anderson, S. K., Handelsman, M. M., & Klevansky, R. (2007). An acculturation model for ethics training: The ethics autobiography and beyond. *Professional Psychology: Research and Practice, 38*, 60–67.

Bernard, J. L., & Jara, C. S. (1986). The failure of clinical psychology graduate students to apply understood ethical principles. *Professional Psychology: Research and Practice, 17*, 313–315.

Bernard, J. M., & Goodyear, R. K. (2004). *Fundamentals of clinical supervision* (3rd ed.). Boston, MA: Pearson Education.

Bernard, J. L., Murphy, M., & Little, M. (1987). The failure of clinical psychologists to apply understood ethical principles. *Professional Psychology: Research and Practice, 18*, 489–491.

Berry, J. W. (1980). Acculturation as varieties of adaptation. In A. M. Padilla (Ed.), *Acculturation: Theory, models, and some new findings* (pp. 9–25). Boulder, CO: Westview Press.

Berry, J. W. (2003). Conceptual approaches to acculturation. In K. M. Chun, P. B. Organista, & G. Marin (Eds.), *Acculturation: Advances in theory, measurement, and applied research* (pp. 17–37). Washington, DC: American Psychological Association.

Berry, J. W., & Kim, U. (1988). Acculturation and mental health. In P. R. Dasen, J. W. Berry, & N. Sartorius (Eds.), *Health and cross-cultural psychology* (pp. 207–236). Newbury Park, NY: Sage.

Berry, J. W., & Sam, D. L. (1997). Acculturation and adaptation. In J. W. Berry, M. H. Segall, & C. Kagitçibasi (Eds.), *Handbook of cross-cultural psychology* (pp. 291–326). Needham Heights, MA: Allyn and Bacon.

Betan, E. J., & Stanton, A. L. (1999). Fostering ethical willingness: Integrating emotional and contextual awareness with rational analysis. *Professional Psychology: Research and Practice, 30*, 295–301.

Birch, J. (1990). The context-setting function of the video "consent" form. *Journal of Family Therapy, 12*, 281–286.

Blumenfeld, W. J., & Raymond, D. (2000). Prejudice and discrimination. In M. Adams, W. J. Blumenfeld, R. Castaneda, H. W. Hackman, M. L. Peters, & X. Zuniga (Eds.), *Readings for diversity and social justice* (pp. 35–49). New York: Routledge.

Bok, S. (1989). *Secrets: On the ethics of concealment and revelation.* New York: Vintage Books.

Braaten, E. B., & Handelsman, M. M. (1997). Client preferences for informed consent information. *Ethics & Behavior, 7,* 311–328.

Braaten, E. B., Otto, S., & Handelsman, M. M. (1993). What do people want to know about psychotherapy? *Psychotherapy, 30,* 565–570.

Branstetter, S. A., & Handelsman, M. M. (2000). Graduate teaching assistants: Ethical training, beliefs, and practices. *Ethics & Behavior, 10,* 27–50.

Bucher, R., & Stelling, J. G. (1977). *Becoming professional.* Beverly Hills: Sage.

Buckley, P., Karasu, T. B., & Charles, E. (1981). Psychotherapists view their personal therapy. *Psychotherapy: Theory, Research, and Practice, 18,* 299–305.

Carifio, M. S., & Hess, A. K. (1987). Who is the ideal supervisor? *Professional Psychology: Research and Practice, 18,* 244–250.

Chauvin, J. C., & Remley, T. P., Jr. (1996). Responding to allegations of unethical conduct. *Journal of Counseling & Development, 74,* 563–568.

Clark, C. R. (1993). Social responsibility ethics: Doing right, doing good, doing well. *Ethics and Behavior, 3,* 303–328.

Corey, C., Corey, M. S., & Callanan, P. (2007). *Issues and ethics in the helping professions* (7th ed.). Belmont, CA: Brooks Cole.

Cornish, J., Kitchener, K. S., & Barnett, J. (2008, August). Supervisor and supervisee ethical expectations – What goes on behind closed doors? Paper presentation at the 116th Annual Convention of the American Psychological Association, Boston, MA.

Cottone, R. R., & Claus, R. E. (2000). Ethical decision-making models: A review of the literature. *Journal of Counseling and Development, 78,* 275–283.

Cottone, R. R., & Tarvydas, V. M. (2007). *Counseling ethics and decision making* (3rd ed.). Upper Saddle River, NJ: Pearson Merrill Prentice Hall.

Cottone, R. R., Tarvydas, V., & Claus, R. E. (2007). Ethical decision-making process. In R. R. Cottone & V. M. Tarvydas (Eds.), *Counseling ethics and decision making* (3rd ed.). Upper Saddle River, NJ: Pearson Merrill Prentice Hall.

Coyne, J. C., & Widiger, T. A. (1978). Toward a participatory model of psychotherapy. *Professional Psychology, 9,* 700–701.

Deutsch, C. J. (1984). Self-reported sources of stress among psychotherapists. *Professional Psychology: Research and Practice, 15,* 835–845.

Driscoll, J. M. (1992). Keeping covenants and confidences sacred: One point of view. *Journal of Counseling and Development, 70,* 704–708.

Ellis, M. V. (1991). Critical incidents in clinical supervision and in supervisor supervision: Assessing supervisory issues. *Journal of Counseling Psychology, 38,* 342–349.

Furman, R. (2005). White male privilege in the context of my life. In S. K. Anderson & V. A. Middleton (Eds.), *Explorations in privilege, oppression and discrimination* (pp. 25–29). Belmont, CA: Thomson Brooks/Cole.

Gilley, J. W., Anderson, S. K., & Gilley, A. (2008). Ethics in human resources. In S. Quatro (Ed.), *Executive ethics: Ethical dilemmas and challenges for the C-suite*. Charlotte, NC: Information Age Publishing.

Glaser, R. D., & Thorpe, J. S. (1986). Unethical intimacy: A survey of sexual contact and advances between psychology educators and female graduate students. *American Psychologist, 41*, 43–51.

Gottlieb, M. C. (1993). Avoiding exploitive dual relationships: A decision-making model. *Psychotherapy, 30*, 41–48.

Grater, H. A. (1985). Stages in psychotherapy supervision: From therapy skills to skilled therapist. *Professional Psychology: Research and Practice, 16*, 605–610.

Gutheil, T. G., & Gabbard, G. O. (1993). The concept of boundaries in clinical practice: Theoretical and risk-management dimensions. *American Journal of Psychiatry, 150*, 188–196.

Hammel, G. A., Olkin, R., & Taube, D. O. (1996). Student-educator sex in clinical and counseling psychology doctoral training. *Professional Psychology: Research and Practice, 27*, 93–97.

Handelsman, M. M. (1987). Confidentiality: The ethical baby in the legal bathwater. *Journal of Applied Rehabilitation Counseling, 18*(4), 33–34.

Handelsman, M. M. (2001a). Accurate and effective informed consent. In E. R. Welfel & R. E. Ingersoll (Eds.), *The mental health desk reference* (pp. 453–458). New York: Wiley.

Handelsman, M. M. (2001b). Learning to become ethical. In S. Walfish & A. K. Hess (Eds.), *Succeeding in graduate school: The career guide for psychology students* (pp. 189–202). Mahwah, NJ: Lawrence Erlbaum.

Handelsman, M. M., & Galvin, M. D. (1988). Facilitating informed consent for outpatient psychotherapy: A suggested written format. *Professional Psychology: Research and Practice, 19*, 223–225.

Handelsman, M. M., Gottlieb, M. C., & Knapp, S. (2005). Training ethical psychologists: An acculturation model. *Professional Psychology: Research and Practice, 36*, 59–65.

Handelsman, M. M., Knapp, S., & Gottlieb, M. C. (2002). Positive ethics. In C. R. Snyder & S. J. Lopez (Eds.), *Handbook of positive psychology* (pp. 731–744). New York: Oxford University Press.

Handelsman, M. M., Knapp, S., & Gottlieb, M. C. (in press). Positive ethics: Themes and variations. In C. R. Snyder & S. J. Lopez (Eds.), *Handbook of positive psychology* (2nd ed.). New York: Oxford University Press.

Harrar, W. R., VandeCreek, L., & Knapp, S. (1990). Ethical and legal aspects of clinical supervision. *Professional Psychology: Research and Practice, 21*, 37–41.

Haynes, R., Corey, G., & Moulton, P. (2003). *Clinical supervision in the helping professions: A practical guide*. Pacific Grove, CA: Brooks/Cole.

Henderson, C. E., Cawyer, C. S., & Watkins, C. E. (1999). A comparison of student and supervisor perceptions of effective practicum supervision. *Clinical Supervisor, 18*, 47–74.

Holloway, E. L. (1992). Supervision: A way of learning and teaching. In S. D. Brown & R. W. Lent (Eds.), *Handbook of counseling psychology* (2nd ed., pp. 177–214). New York: Wiley.

Jensen, P. S., Josephson, A. M., & Frey, J. (1989). Informed consent as a framework for treatment: Ethical and therapeutic concerns. *American Journal of Psychotherapy, 43*, 378–386.

Jevne, P., & Williams, D. R. (1998). *When dreams don't work: Professional caregivers and burnout.* Amityville, NY: Baywood.

Jordan, A., & Meara, N. (1990). Ethics and the professional practice of psychologists: The role of virtues and principles. *Professional Psychology: Theory and Practice, 21*, 106–114.

Kennard, B. D., Stewart, S. M., & Gluck, M. R. (1987). The supervisory relationship: Variables contributing to positive versus negative experiences. *Professional Psychology: Research and Practice, 18*, 172–175.

Kitchener, K. S. (2000). *Foundations of ethical practice in research and teaching in psychology.* Mahwah, NJ: Lawrence Erlbaum.

Knapp, S. J., & VandeCreek, L. D. (2006). *Practical ethics for psychologists: A positive approach.* Washington, DC: American Psychological Association.

Koocher, G. P. (1979). Credentialing in psychology: Close encounters with competence? *American Psychologist, 34*, 696–702.

Kramer, S. A. (1986). The termination process in open-ended psychotherapy: Guidelines for clinical practice. *Psychotherapy, 23*, 526–531.

Kuther, T. L. (2003). Promoting positive ethics: An interview with Mitchell M. Handelsman. *Teaching of Psychology, 30*, 339–343.

Ladany, N., Ellis, M. V., & Friedlander, M. L. (1999). The supervisory working alliance, trainee self-efficacy, and satisfaction with supervision. *Journal of Counseling & Development, 77*, 447–455.

Lazarus, A. A., & Zur, O. (2002). *Dual relationships and psychotherapy.* New York: Springer.

Liddle, B. J. (2005). Tales from the heart of Dixie: Using white privilege to fight racism. In S. K. Anderson & V. A. Middleton (Eds.), *Explorations in privilege, oppression and discrimination* (pp. 171–176). Belmont, CA: Thomson Brooks/ Cole.

Lo, K. (2005). Seeing through another lens. In S. K. Anderson & V. A. Middleton (Eds.), *Explorations in privilege, oppression and discrimination* (pp. 49–52). Belmont, CA: Thomson Brooks/Cole.

Loganbill, C., Hardy, E., & Delworth, U. (1983). Supervision: A conceptual model. *Counseling Psychologist, 10*, 3–42.

Loomis, C. (2005). Understanding and experiencing class privilege. In S. K. Anderson & V. A. Middleton (Eds.), *Explorations in privilege, oppression and discrimination* (pp. 31–39). Belmont, CA: Thomson Brooks/Cole.

Lustig, M., & Koester, J. (1999). *Intercultural competence: Interpersonal communication across cultures* (3rd ed.). New York: Addison Wesley Longman.

Maki, D. R., & Bernard, J. M. (2007). The ethics of clinical supervision. In R. R. Cottone and V. M. Tarvydas (Eds.). *Counseling ethics and decision making* (pp. 347–368).

Martino, C. (2001, August). Secrets of successful supervision: Graduate students' preferences and experiences with effective and ineffective supervision. In J. E. Barnett (Chair), *Secrets of successful supervision – Clinical and ethical issues*. Symposium conducted at the 109th Annual Convention of the American Psychological Association, San Francisco, CA.

McIntosh, P. (1990, Winter). White privilege: Unpacking the invisible knapsack. *Independent School, 49*(2), 31–36.

McIntosh, P. (2000). White privilege and male privilege: A personal account of coming to see correspondences through work in women's studies. In A. Minas (Ed.), *Gender basics: Feminist perspectives on women and men* (2nd ed., pp. 30–38). Belmont, CA: Wadsworth/Thomas Learning.

Meara, N., Schmidt, L., & Day, J. (1996). Principles and virtues: A foundation for ethical decisions, policies, and character. *The Counseling Psychologist, 24*, 4–77.

Megivern, D. (2005). Supposed to know better. In S. K. Anderson & V. A. Middleton (Eds.), *Explorations in privilege, oppression and discrimination* (pp. 17–29). Belmont, CA: Thomson Brooks/Cole.

Myers, J. E., Sweeney, T. J., & Witmer, J. M. (2000). The wheel of wellness counseling for wellness: A holistic model. *Journal of Counseling and Development, 78*(3), 251–266.

Nagy, T. F. (2000). *Ethics in plain English*. Washington, DC: American Psychological Association.

National Association of Social Workers. (1999). *Code of ethics*. Washington, DC: Author.

O'Reilly, R. (1987). The transfer syndrome. *Canadian Journal of Psychiatry, 32*, 674–678.

Peterson, C., & Seligman, M. E. P. (2004). *Character strengths and virtues: A handbook and classification*. New York: Oxford University Press.

Pomerantz, A., & Handelsman, M. M. (2004). Informed consent revisited: An updated written question format. *Professional Psychology: Research and Practice, 35*, 201–205.

Pope, K. S., Sonne, J. L., & Greene, B. (2006). *What therapists don't talk about and why*. Washington, DC: American Psychological Association.

Pope, K. S., & Vetter, V. A. (1992). Ethical dilemmas encountered by members of the APA: A national survey. *American Psychologist, 47*, 397–411.

Rest, J. R. (1983). Morality. In P. Mussen (General Ed.), and J. Flavell & E. Markman (Vol. Eds.), *Handbook of child psychology: Vol. IV. Cognitive development*. New York: Wiley.

Rest, J. R. (1984). Research on moral development: Implications for training counseling psychologists. *Counseling Psychologist 12*(3), 19–29.

Rest, J. R. (1986). *Moral development: Advances in research and theory*. New York: Praeger.

Rest, J. R. (1994). Background: Theory and research. In J. R. Rest & D. Narváez (Eds.), *Moral development in the professions: Psychology and applied ethics* (pp. 1–26). Hillsdale, NJ: Lawrence Erlbaum.

Rest, J. R., & Narváez, D. (Eds.). (1994). *Moral development in the professions: Psychology and applied ethics*. Hillsdale, NJ: Lawrence Erlbaum.

Rice, N. M., & Follette, V. M. (2003). The termination and referral of clients. In W. O'Donohue & K. Ferguson (Eds.), *Handbook of professional ethics for psychologists: Issues, questions, and controversies* (pp. 147–166). Thousand Oaks, CA: Sage.

Sherry, P. (1991). Ethical issues in the conduct of supervision. *The Counseling Psychologist, 19*, 566–585.

Siegel, M. (1979). Privacy, ethics, and confidentiality. *Professional Psychology: Research and Practice, 10*, 249–258.

Skovholt, T. M. (2001). *The resilient practitioner: Burnout prevention and self-care strategies for counselors, therapists, teachers, and health professionals*. Boston: Allyn & Bacon.

Stoltenberg, C., & Delworth, U. (1987). *Supervising counselors and therapists: A developmental approach*. San Francisco: Jossey Bass.

Sue, D. W., & Sue, D. (2003). *Counseling the culturally different: Theory and practice* (4th ed.). New York: Wiley.

Sullivan, T., Martin, W. L., Jr., & Handelsman, M. M. (1993). Practical benefits of an informed consent procedure. *Professional Psychology: Research and Practice, 24*, 160–163.

Tarasoff v. Regents of the University of California, 529 P.2d 553 (Cal. 1974), 551 P.2d 334, 331 (Cal. 1976).

Tatum, B. D. (1999). Lighting candles in the dark: One black woman's response to white antiracist narratives. In C. Clark and J. O'Donnell (Eds.), *Becoming and unbecoming white: Owning and disowning a racial identity* (pp. 56–63). Westport, CT: Bergin and Garvey.

Thomas, J. T. (2005). Licensing board complaints: Minimizing the impact on the psychologist's defense and clinical practice. *Professional Psychology: Research and Practice, 36*, 426–433.

Tuason, M. T. (2005). Deprivations and privileges we all have. In S. K. Anderson & V. A. Middleton (Eds.), *Explorations in privilege, oppression and discrimination*. (pp. 41–47). Belmont, CA: Thomson Brooks/Cole.

Veatch, R. M., & Sollitto, S. (1976). Medical ethics teaching: Report of a national medical school survey. *Journal of the American Medical Association, 235,* 1030–1033.

Watkins, C. E. (1995). Psychotherapy supervision in the 1990s: Some observations and reflections. *American Journal of Psychotherapy, 49,* 568–581.

Welfel, E. R. (2002). *Ethics in counseling and psychotherapy: Standards, research, and emerging issues* (2nd ed.). Belmont, CA: Thomson Brooks/Cole.

Welfel, E. R. (2006). *Ethics in counseling and psychotherapy: Standards, research, and emerging issues* (3rd ed.). Belmont, CA: Thomson Brooks/Cole.

Wise, E. H. (2007). Informed consent: Complexities and meanings. *Professional Psychology: Research and Practice, 38,* 182–183.

Wulf, J., & Nelson, M. L. (2000). Experienced psychologists' recollections of internship supervision and its contributions to their development. *Clinical Supervisor, 19,* 123–145.

Author Index

Subject Index

.

Printed and bound by CPI Group (UK) Ltd, Croydon, CR0 4YY

27/10/2024

14580369-0002